Computer Literacy
in Human Services

Computer Literacy in Human Services

Richard Reinoehl
Thomas Hanna
Editors

The Haworth Press
New York • London

Computer Literacy in Human Services has also been published as *Computers in Human Services*, Volume 6 1990.

The Haworth Press, Inc., 10 Alice Street, Binghamton, NY 13904-1580
EUROSPAN/Haworth, 3 Henrietta Street, London WC2E 8LU England

Library of Congress Cataloging-in-Publication Data

Computer literacy in human services / Richard Reinoehl, Thomas Hanna, editors.
    p. cm.
    Also published as Computers in human services, v. 6, 1990.
    ISBN 0-86656-866-2 (alk. paper)
    1. Human services—Data processing. 2. Computer literacy. I. Reinoehl, Richard. II. Hanna, Thomas. III. Computers in human services.
HV29.2.C66   1990
361'.0028'5—dc20
                                                     89-71738
                                                        CIP

Computer Literacy in Human Services

CONTENTS

SECTION IV: ADVANCED APPLICATIONS: INFLUENCING THE FUTURE OF HUMAN SERVICES

EXTENDED TABLE OF CONTENTS

ABOUT THE EDITORS

Richard Reinoehl is Director of the Human Development Consortium, Inc., located in Ithaca, New York.

Thomas Hanna is Program Development Coordinator for the Family Life Development Center, Department of Human Development and Family Studies at New York State College of Human Ecology of Cornell University in Ithaca, New York.

Introduction

This volume defines and exemplifies computer literacy in human services, addressing the perspectives of both practitioners and scholars. The volume was not designed as a primer for individuals who are taking their first step into either computers or human services. Other publications exist which accomplish those tasks. Rather, it is intended for those who already have come to recognize that the computer will be playing an important part in the future of human services and who want to prepare further for their role in it.

The first section offers a detailed definitional and issue-oriented perspective on computer literacy that provides a cognitive structure for sorting and assessing much of the work published on computer use in human services. Readers may also find the definitional approach useful for interpretation of the balance of articles in the present volume. It is important to point out, however, that the other sections have not been organized to adhere to the structural aspects of the definitional model, although they do move generally from an "entry point" of computer utilization to the current frontiers of computer literacy in the human services.

The second section addresses the creative use of existing commercial software in solving human services problems. The third section provides a series of articles describing the development—by human service professionals—of software applications specifically designed for human service settings. The final section explores the frontier of computer technology in human services, where the highest levels of ability are needed for developing the potentials of such applications.

Throughout we have selected contributions that span a broad range of computer applications in the human services. However, there are areas of computer uses in human service that we have not addressed. Therefore, we urge the reader to look elsewhere for information on topics such as electronic networking, computer assisted instruction, dynamic modeling, and hyper media. Nevertheless, most readers should find sufficient material here for increasing their own computer literacy in human services.

Richard Reinoehl
Thomas Hanna
Editors

SECTION I:
INTRODUCING AND STABILIZING THE CONCEPT OF COMPUTER LITERACY

Defining Computer Literacy in Human Services

Richard Reinoehl
Thomas Hanna

KEYWORDS. Computers, computer literacy, child protection, child neglect, child abuse

SUMMARY. Computer literacy in human services is defined as an intersection of *both* computer and human services abilities. With different levels of ability possible, a matrix is created which can be used to operationally define computer literacy within any area of human service practice. Child protective work is used to demonstrate the utility of this definitional approach. Various issues within computer literacy are also discussed.

Richard Reinoehl is Director of the Human Development Consortium, Inc., a computer consulting group working with human service organizations and institutions of higher learning, 24 Uptown Village, Ithaca, NY 14850. He is a past faculty of the Social Work Program, University of Wisconsin, Superior.

Thomas Hanna is the Program Development Coordinator for the Family Life Development Center, Human Development and Family Studies, New York State College of Human Ecology, Cornell University, Ithaca, NY 14853-4401.

INTRODUCTION

Human service professionals are generally aware of the expanding utility of computers and the accompanying need for computer literacy. Indeed, individuals and organizations have invested substantial resources to learn more about computers and to develop computer enhanced work environments.

This fact, combined with continuing innovation, is providing an array of exciting possibilities for all areas of human service. Computer applications have thus far included new tools for clinical assessment (Johnson, 1984; Schwartz, 1984; Merrell, 1985; Nurius, 1990), direct therapy (Allen, 1984; Clarke & Schoech, 1984; Figley, 1985), case management (Blazyk, Wimberley & Crawford, 1987), administration (Romano, Conklin & Fisher 1985; Slavin, 1981; Korte, 1990), training (Saka, 1985; Lynett, 1985), evaluation (Trochim, 1985; Gray 1986; Yonai, 1986; Hug, 1990) and policy and planning (Flynn, 1987). Among the categories of software available for use are relational databases, spreadsheets, idea processors, dynamic modeling programs, expert and decision support systems, electronic mail and bulletin boards, hyper media and desktop publishing systems.

Unfortunately, with all this potential at hand, some of the most basic efforts at computerization continue to result in frustration, and in systems which are more costly or less effective than desired. Additionally, these thwarted attempts only infrequently find their way into the professional literature, where there could be an analysis of the reasons for difficulties. More often, knowledge of these negative experiences emerge through observation and discussion with colleagues.

Among such cases known to us are:

1. A community mental health center which purchased a $60,000 minicomputer for purposes of clinical assessment, not realizing that similar software also ran on an inexpensive microcomputer.

2. A family counseling center which purchased a microcomputer for several thousand dollars, and over the next three years spent ten times that amount in staff and consulting time in order to program the computer to meet organizational needs.

The manual system was finally resurrected because the computer was printing inaccurate amounts on checks.[1]

As we compliment those who have succeeded in developing and using successful new computer applications, it would be equally easy to blame organizational decision makers or consultants for inadequate or "problem" computer systems. However, there is also the possibility of a more important professional consideration: that there is no clearly marked body of knowledge and skills which can consistently guide the application of computers in human services. Thus, individuals who attempt to specify or design computer systems for human services can unknowingly be deficient in their understanding of either computers *or* human services.

Omissions in either ability can, and often do, result in acquisition of computer systems that fall quite short of their intended purpose. Therefore, if one is to avoid these pitfalls, it is important to determine which abilities are necessary for computer competence in human services. It is this question of ability that is at the core of the ambiguity and general confusion that exists in attempts to define computer literacy.

DEFINING COMPUTER LITERACY

Our definition and its subsequent use is based in two assumptions. The first is that computer literacy is not computer science, but is computer ability *in relationship* to ability in a professional or academic area. Thus, computer literacy within a field, such as human services, is a relatively unique collection of intersections of computer and human services abilities.

The second assumption is that there are differing levels of ability, and these levels can be divided into three general categories: (1) a beginning awareness, (2) proficiency, and (3) creative development. Beginning awareness is the level an individual occupies as he or she is learning the concepts, theories and skills involved within a professional pursuit. At the level of proficiency, an individual would have an integration and mastery of these theories and skills; this is a

---

1. The examples cited come from confidential discussions and interviews with agency directors and employees.

professional level where an individual evaluates a situation and selects from his or her repertoire the most appropriate action(s). The highest level, creative development, involves inspiration — the making of hitherto unmade connections that result in new constructs useful in extending the practice or the conceptual/theoretical basis of a profession (Reinoehl, Iroff & McLennan, 1988).

Thus, if we agree that computer literacy involves an intersection of computer ability with professional expertise, a general definition emerges for human service. That is:

> *Computer literacy in human services is the ability to use or develop computer applications competently within the context of human service theory or practice.*

Using computer and human services ability as dimensions, this general definition can be expanded into a three-by-three matrix (Figure I) for the systematic development of operational definitions. In fact, we can envision the matrix as a conceptual window which rotates on the "computer abilities" axis through the epistemological space comprising human services. Different abilities appear in the window as it rotates through each of the varying roles and domains of the field. When we pause in the rotation to focus attention on a particular area, it acts to determine the specific abilities of that area (ibid).

AN EXAMPLE IN HUMAN SERVICE

We could use the matrix at a level of generality that would provide a definition applicable to a variety of human service occupations. However, we chose to work at an operational level and select a specific area of focus: casework in child abuse and neglect (child protection).

To provide the unique coincidence of child protective expertise with computer abilities is not a simple task. Although there is some documentation of this interstice (Schwab, Bruce & McRoy, 1986), the full breadth of innovative computer applications developed in the last few years is not addressed in the literature. At the same time, a comprehensive examination of all possible intersections would occupy more space than we have available. Therefore, we

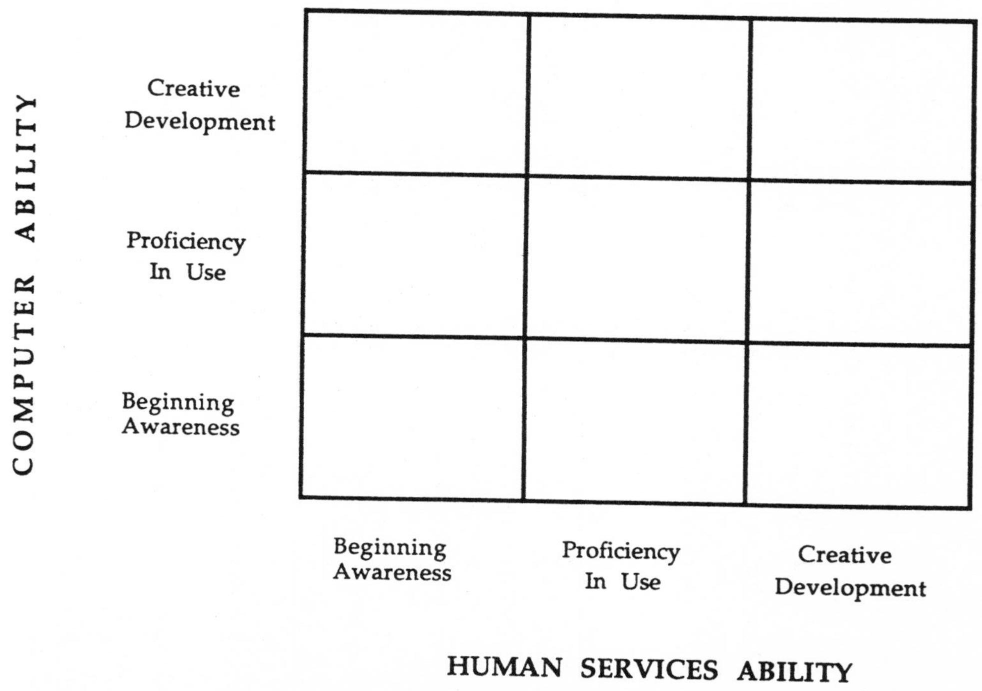

HUMAN SERVICES ABILITY

FIGURE I. Computer Literacy Matrix

7

provide selected examples for the purpose of illustration. Since not all readers will be familiar with this area of human service, we first review some of the abilities which constitute different levels of competence in child protection. For these levels we suggest:

- *A beginning awareness* includes the range from no knowledge or ability to a functional competence in understanding local child protection laws, local resources, the roles (investigation, assessment and case management) played by a child protective worker, and sufficient skill to apply this knowledge. In most states the caseworker would be a college graduate, but would not necessarily have a social work degree or any formal education or experience in the human services.

- At a level of *proficiency*, a child protective worker would not only have achieved a mastery of the above, but would have developed strong analytical and evaluative powers. These abilities would provide the capacity to manage many active cases while maintaining a low "miss rate" on assessing the risk of a child, and a high success rate on families that "make it." Such a worker would also be aware of differing models of intervention, their possible strength and weaknesses, and could assess which would be most appropriate for a given situation. Post-graduate training in the field would generally be associated with this level of ability.

- *Creative development* in child abuse work would involve the ability to define and inspire new methods, models or theories affecting traditional case management, especially in problematic arenas such as chronic neglect, severe physical abuse, familial sexual abuse, emotional degradation, and drug abuse and AIDS related forms of maltreatment. Creativity could also involve the development of new analytical techniques for determining the presence or absence of child abuse or neglect, or assessing risk to a child.

With these distinctions in mind, we move to generating the differing intersections of computer and child protective abilities. For consistency we repeat the pattern used in describing child protective ability, i.e., beginning awareness, proficiency, and creative development, but this time repeated in conjunction with each of the three levels of computer ability, starting with beginning computer awareness. We provide some examples that are specific to child protective work and others that also apply to other areas of human service. Figure II shows how some of the examples would appear graphically in the computer literacy matrix, but due to space limitations there is only one example use per cell. It should be kept in mind that these examples are attempts to give the "flavor" of a cell, rather than to fully define each cell and its boundaries.

Beginning Computer Awareness

At this level a computer would provide elementary tools matched to child protective abilities.

- **Beginning Awareness in Child Protection:** The abilities in this cell would include: *use a word processor to take notes, or to modify form letters for individual clients; access, fill in, and save completed forms that appear on a computer screen; and, use menu selections to receive reports from a database.*

- **Proficiency in Child Protective Practice:** The abilities in this cell would include: *use a word processor to write a report comparing differing models of child/family intervention; use a decision support system designed to assist in referral; and, evaluate work load to determine possible usefulness of an existing database template designed for tracking cases.*

- **Creative Development in Child Protection:** The abilities in this cell would include: *use a word processor to write a publishable article advancing a re-definition of the role of the child protective worker; use a time-resource planning package to map "critical intervention" pathways for various child abuse situations.*

Proficiency in Using Computers

At this level a worker can bring wide-ranging computer resources to bear on tasks and problems faced on the job.

ABILITY IN CHILD PROTECTION

COMPUTER ABILITY	Beginning Awareness	Proficiency In Use	Creative Development
Creative Development	Develop time management software that could be useful in child protective work	Design a DSS for assisting a child protective unit in adhering to practice standards for child protective investigations	Design a dynamic modeling program to facilitate development of new assessment and treatment methods
Proficiency In Use	Evaluate authoring programs for use in translating an existing training curriculum on child abuse & neglect into a CAI package	Determine whether a free-form database package, hypertext program, or idea processor would best aid in structuring case notes	Develop a child evaluation/tracking system using the most appropriate database management program
Beginning Awareness	Use a word processor to take notes or to modify a form letter for individual clients	Use a word processor to write client progress and summary reports	Use a word processor to write a publishable article advancing a re-definition of the role of child protective worker

FIGURE II. Computer Literacy in Child Protection

- **Beginning Awareness in Child Protection:** The abilities in this cell would include: *evaluate which authoring program might be best for translating an existing training curriculum on child abuse and neglect into a Computer Assisted Instruction (CAI) package, and; evaluate time-management programs for potential use in structuring work schedules.*

- **Proficiency in Child Protection:** The abilities in this cell would include: *determine which word processor would best meet the needs for reports, letters, and textual data sharing with co-workers; determine whether use of a free-form database package, hypertext program, idea processor, or a combination of software, would best aid in structuring extensive case notes, and; determine which database might best be applied to tracking and assessing family treatment.*

- **Creative Development in Child Protection:** The abilities in this cell would include: *develop a child evaluation/tracking system using a database management program; use existing software to develop a child abuse decision support system, and use a dynamic modeling program to compare intervention models for family child abuse and develop case-appropriate modifications of such models.*

Creative Development in Using Computers

In these cells an individual, or more likely a team of individuals, would use the computer to create resources to solve challenging problems — even problems that were previously ill-defined.

- **Beginning Awareness in Child Protection:** The abilities in this cell would include: *use a high level computer language, such as Pascal or C, to translate an existing protocol for risk assessment in child abuse and neglect into a Computer Assisted Risk Evaluation package; and, develop a generalized time management program that might be useful in child protective work.*

- **Proficiency in Child Protection:** The abilities in this cell would include: *design a decision support system for assisting a child protective unit in adhering to practice standards for child protective investigations; and, develop a Local Area Net-*

work (LAN) useful for data sharing and team assessment among child protective workers.

- **Creative Development in Child Protection:** (We do not expect many developments to occur soon at these altitudes.) The abilities in this cell would include: *develop a concept mapping program designed to facilitate brain storming for new assessment and treatment methods; develop a multitasking information management system for child protective services that includes (1) service-wide data gathering and analysis, (2) self-assessment utilities for individual workers, and (3) district-level caseload risk analyses; and, a "situation room" program that allows for team assessment of present high risk cases based on past casework experience.*

One can observe that some examples used for the intersections of computer and child protection abilities are not far from what has already been accomplished or planned for resolving complicated problems in human services. A statewide effort at developing and implementing a decision support system for offering home-based services to the disabled elderly (Pruger, 1988) provides just one example. Nonetheless, the real world instances of the linking of higher level computer power and difficult service delivery problems are still rare. Thus, although some of these examples represent a certain confessed extravagance of imagination, they also represent a reasonable projection that tests the conceptual utility of the computer literacy matrix, and makes note of what is possible through a more thorough utilization of existing computer technology.

This "test" of the matrix is additionally offered as an example exercise for those interested in defining and promoting computer literacy in their own areas of human service. Although refinement of these concepts and their relationships could add some incremental benefit, its current status provides enough form and consistency that one could use the matrix to develop proposals of computer literacy standards within a specific area of practice. We assume that a comprehensive definition of computer literacy in child protection, for example, would best be undertaken by the professionals who have already achieved a high proficiency of computer literacy in the field of child abuse and neglect.

DISCUSSION

The preceding definition and example demonstrate the utility of the matrix as a definitional tool. However, there are some important relationships that may not be initially apparent and would benefit from further elaboration. Of these, the first involves the double meaning of literacy.

A discerning reader may have noticed a difference in terms between the definition of computer literacy and the matrix, i.e., the use of "competently" in the former, and "proficiency" in the latter. At first this may seem unnecessary and confusing, as the use of the same term in both places would more clearly show a relationship between the general definition and the computer literacy matrix. However, the difference between being competent (having an adequate ability) and proficient (having an advanced ability) is an important distinction in literacy issues. That is, in common usage — such as is found in most dictionaries — the term "literate" has two meanings and can refer to either (1) functional literacy, the ability to read and write, or (2) to be well versed or polished (proficient) in literature and creative writing.

When applied to computers, we can say that functional computer literacy is the basic level of computer ability that enables an individual to adequately use a computer in the performance of his or her occupational role(s). It involves such abilities as knowing how to turn a computer (or terminal) on and off, how to perform file and disk manipulations — such as accessing, saving and copying, and the use of one or more application programs.

Computer use at this level is generally routine and tends to be based on rote learning. A functional literacy can be obtained through a few days of training followed by several weeks or months of practice. When discretionary decisions occur at this level, they are usually between options within a program (using a tab function vs. re-setting the margin) or between program types (deciding between a word processor and a spreadsheet to develop an alpha/numeric table). Because individuals can reach an initial level of functional literacy with a relatively small base of knowledge, this group of abilities involves the greater part of the beginning awareness level of computers.

The higher level of literacy involves proficiency, an advanced achievement of expertise which, within most areas of human service, would be the level associated with the standards for professional accreditation. At this level, an individual would have a broad base of knowledge and skills which transcends the needs of a specific work environment. Such an individual would be able to evaluate a variety of computer technologies to determine the most appropriate for a given situation. For example, an individual at this level would not only be able to use an on-the-job database (functional computer literacy), but could accurately evaluate a range of commercially available database programs to determine which might better meet his or her professional needs. In another example, if an individual wished to determine how a computer could assist in organizing extensive case notes, he or she would first assess differing types of hardware and software, such as, idea processors, text oriented databases, hypertext programs, etc., for applicability, and then proceed to evaluate which, within the selected type, would be the best choice. (Although, the applicability of a final computer product would also vary on the level of the human service experience and ability involved.)

These explanations not only demonstrate the difference between the functional/beginning awareness level and the proficiency level in computer literacy (see Figure III), but also shows the importance of the proficiency level as a baseline of ability important in achieving a high quality outcome in creative development. Of course, this does not necessarily mean that creativity at a lower level of ability will always result in a poorly developed product, or that a proficiency level will always result in a high quality product — variables other than individual competence, such as organizational support and external resources, are involved. Rather, it emphasizes that with other conditions being equal, the higher the ability levels involved, the more likely a desired result will occur.

The second issue involves the relationship of abilities within matrix cells to the individuals who may embody them. It is not difficult to find examples of individuals whose abilities fall within a specific cell or cells. It is tempting, therefore, to imagine that all individuals will have abilities that fit snugly within specific cells. However, we wish to stress that this is not the case. For instance, an individual

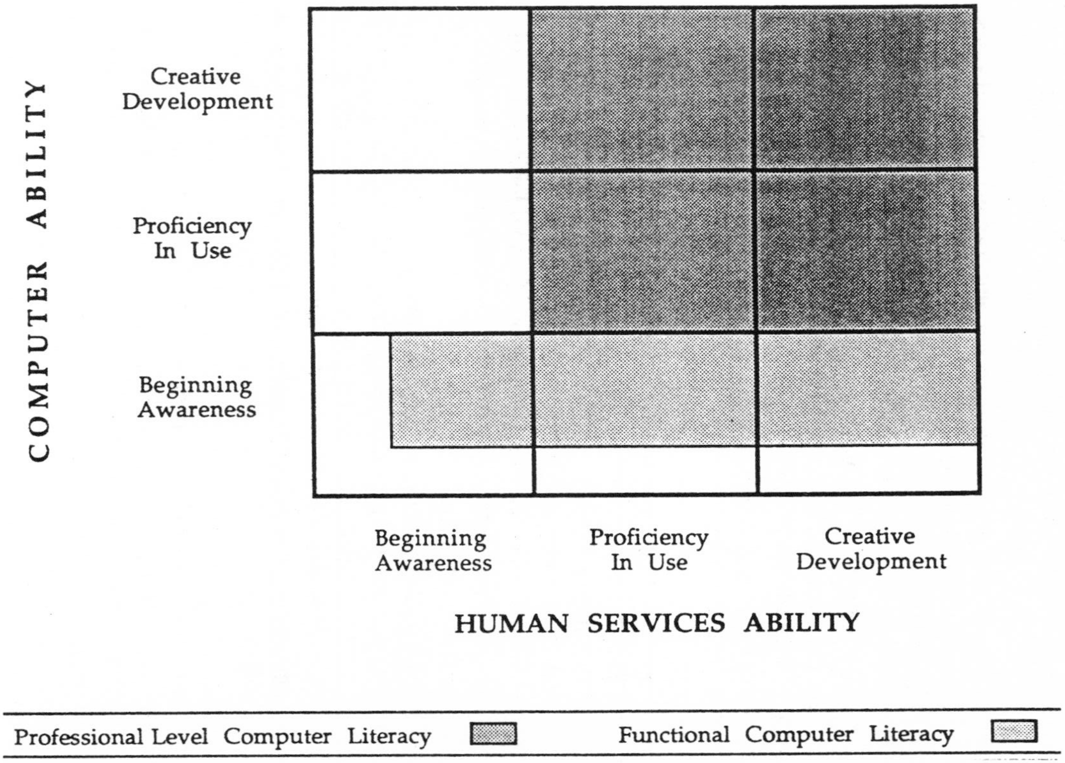

HUMAN SERVICES ABILITY

COMPUTER ABILITY

Creative Development — Proficiency In Use — Beginning Awareness

Beginning Awareness — Proficiency In Use — Creative Development

Professional Level Computer Literacy   Functional Computer Literacy

FIGURE III. Professional vs. Functional Computer Literacy

15

who has extensive experience with a variety of word processors, but limited experience with other types of software would be at a proficiency level in regard to word processing, but no more than functionally literate in other areas.

Another instance of this issue involves the highest level of computer ability, particularly the cell at the upper right corner. Although it is possible for one individual to be accomplished at a high professional level in two fields, and to be simultaneously creative in both, it is unlikely to occur with any great frequency. Rather, we expect that the exemplification of these intersections will be found most often in the form of collaborations.

The third issue is the relationship of computer programming to computer literacy. In this volume, Flynn (1990), reviews the basic arguments for both sides of the debate over whether literacy is predicated on mastery of programming languages. Because of the historic emphasis on computer hardware, the binary numbering system, Boolean logic, etc., the ability to program in a high level language has been a frequent stereotype of computer literacy. However, the issue takes on another dimension if consideration is given to how rapid technological advances have altered the conditions which gave rise to this thinking.

In this regard, there are three key factors which have influenced our perspective. Initially, there were few application programs available in human services, and knowing how to program was therefore an essential ability for using a computer. However, due to the rapidly changing nature of the computer field and the plethora of application programs which now exist, programming in a high level language is now no more necessary to computer literacy in human services than is the knowledge of how to design a digital circuit.

Another factor is that many applications now blend so thoroughly the ability to "enter and retrieve information" with the ability to "design" methods of managing that information that the old distinctions between programming as a discreet skill and using packaged applications are dissolving or have disappeared. For instance, a spreadsheet user who is using macros to create a new application is actually engaged in a form of programming.

Further, the ability to program can vary over a considerable range, and taking an introductory course in a given computer language does not make someone either computer literate or a good programmer. Programming at a level of beginning awareness can be useful for simple tasks; but if an individual were to use this elementary programming knowledge in an attempt to create a relational database for a human service agency, it would prove to be a costly undertaking.

Knowledge *about* programming with a high level language is important at the highest points of proficiency with computers, but knowing *how* to program in a high level language seems less important for computer literacy in human services than the ability to communicate or collaborate with a professional programmer. Similarly, the ability to program well in a computer language should not be rated above some of the other computer oriented abilities: such as the ability to compare different programming languages to determine the one most appropriate to the task at hand; or the ability to perform a competent system analysis in a human service organization.

Thus, we conclude that although knowledge of programming can be included in a continuum of literacy, it is far from being the quintessential definer of computer literacy in human services. More important for literacy in human services is the ability to (1) understand the structures and dynamics of information in regard to human service needs, and (2) determine how these needs can be addressed through the most cost-effective application of computer technology.

The last issue concerns the relationship of computer literacy to human service organizations. There is a considerable analysis that needs to occur regarding the ramifications for organizational roles, and because of its extensive nature this will need to be the subject of another work. An important contribution to such a discussion, analyzing the reward system in human service organizations and the question of *who* shall control the integration of computer technology within human services appears elsewhere in the present volume (Flynn, ibid.). Therefore, rather than give a cursory analysis here, we instead return to the two examples of "problem" computer experiences with which we began.

In the cases described, difficulties developed because of a deficit in knowledge of computers and/or of human services. In the first example, that of a community mental health center, the inhouse "computer expert" was the business manager who had minimal computer training in business courses, and on-the-job training in the financial aspect of human services. His beginning awareness of computers *and* the clinical aspects of human services was simply not sufficient to give him knowledge of the more cost-effective options in computer based client assessment.

In the second example, that of a family counseling center, the "computer expert" was the director, a well trained human service professional whose computer ability derived from his taking an adult education course in BASIC programming. In this situation, his programming ability gave him a beginning awareness of what could be achieved using a computer; unfortunately his computer awareness was not yet at a level of functional literacy. The result was his purchase of a computer whose extraordinarily restrictive architecture would not allow development of the appropriate software — even by a skilled programmer. Thus, the point to be made about these costly attempts is that when an organization engages in computer development, success is much more likely when the developers are proficient in both the relevant human service and in computer use.

CONCLUSION

We began by pointing to problems which have occurred in the use of computers in human services — because of an unperceived gap in a key area of knowledge. Our examples involved experienced professionals who had been given a false sense of confidence that they had been prepared properly to make a key decision for their organizations. As pointed out, this "mistake" is integrally linked to the absence of a functional definition of computer literacy in human services. In essence, if we can't define what abilities are involved, both in computer ability and in human services ability, there is no benchmark against which we can assess ourselves and others as key decisions involving computers are made.

Our attempt to resolve this dilemma has provided both a general definition and a computer literacy matrix which can be used to develop operationally specific definitions in any area of human services. Although we generated some testable examples, we have not yet attempted a comprehensive use of this matrix for a formal proposal of computer literacy within any specific human service domain. This is a next step which can best be accomplished by those with the necessary expertise within each professional area.

We began with a problem, but have ended with a process which may intrinsically stimulate creativity: determining the key computer abilities for an area of human services involves not only a review of current practices, but also a creative exploration of (1) how existing, off-the-shelf technology can be applied in unique and productive ways, and (2) what new applications could be developed to meet specific human service needs. It is this latter aspect which provides the distinction between simply recording the limited abilities currently used in practice, and developing a comprehensive analysis of the abilities which would exist (and benefits which could accrue) if most human service professionals were applying, in their daily practice, the full range of available computer applications.

BIBLIOGRAPHY

Allen, D. H. (1984). The use of computer fantasy games in child therapy. In M. D. Schwartz (Ed.), *Using Computers in Clinical Practice* (pp. 329-334). New York: The Haworth Press.

Blazyk, S., Wimberley, E. T. & Crawford, C. (1987). Computer-based case management for the elderly. *Computers in Human Services*, 2(1/2), 63-77.

Clarke, B. & Schoech, D. (1984). A computer-assisted therapeutic game for adolescents: Initial development and comments. In M. D. Schwartz (Ed.), *Using Computers in Clinical Practice* (pp. 135-153). New York: The Haworth Press.

Figley, C. R. (Ed.). (1985). Computers and family therapy. [Special Issue]. *Journal of Psychotherapy & the Family*, 1(1/2).

Flynn, J. P. (1987). Simulating policy processes through electronic mail. *Computers in Human Services*, 2(1/2), 13-26.

Flynn, J. P. (1990). Issues in the introduction of computer and information technology. Computer Literacy in Human Services. [Special Issue]. *Computers in Human Services*, [This volume].

Gray, P. T. (1986). Desktop publishing. *Evaluation Practice*, 7(3), 4-9.

Hug, R. W. (1990). Statistical Software in the Human Services: Old Frontier or Leading Edge? Computer Literacy in Human Services. [Special Issue]. *Computers in Human Services*, [This volume].

Johnson, J. H. (1984). An overview of computerized testing. In M. D. Schwartz (Ed.), *Using Computers in Clinical Practice* (pp. 131-133). New York: The Haworth Press.

Korte, A. O. (1990). A first order markov model for use in human services. Computer Literacy in Human Services. [Special Issue]. *Computers in Human Services*, [This volume].

Lynett, P. (1985). The current and potential uses of computer assisted interactive videodisc in the education of social workers. *Computers in Human Services*, *1*(4), 75-85.

Merrell, K. W. (1985). Computer use in psychometric assessment: Evaluating benefits and potential problems. *Computers in Human Services*, *1*(3), 59-67.

Nurius, P. (1990). A review of automated assessment. Computer Literacy in Human Services. [Special Issue]. *Computers in Human Services*, [This volume].

Pruger, Robert (1987). Information technology in support of service-delivery decisions. In G. R. Geiss and N. Viswanathan (Eds.), *The Human Edge* (pp. 212-227). New York: The Haworth Press.

Reinoehl, R. L., Iroff, L. D. & McLennan, A. (1988). Computer literacy: A template for definitions. *Collegiate Microcomputer*, *6*(1), 26-32.

Romano, M. D., Conklin, G. S. & Fisher, D. (1985). Designing information systems for hospital work management. *Computers in Human Services*, *1*(3), 47-58.

Saka, T. T. (1985). Computer work skills training for persons with developmental disabilities. *Computers in Human Services*, *1*(4), 39-51.

Schwab, A. J., Bruce, M. E. & McRoy, R. G. (1986). Using computer technology in child placement decisions. *Social Casework: The Journal of Contemporary Social Work*, *67*(6) 359-68.

Schwartz, M. D. (1984). Review of a probabilistic system for identifying suicide attempts. In M. D. Schwartz (Ed.), *Using Computers in Clinical Practice* (pp. 213-14). New York: The Haworth Press.

Slavin, S. (1981). Applying computers in social service & mental health agencies: A guide to selecting equipment, procedures and strategies. [Special Issue]. *Administration in Social Work*, *5*(3/4).

Trochim, W. M. K. & Davis, J. E. (1985). Computer simulation of human service program evaluations. *Computers in Human Services*, *1*(4), 17-38.

Yonai, B. (1986). Project management software. *Evaluation Practice*, *7*(4), 41-51.

Issues in the Introduction of Computer and Information Technology in Human Services

John P. Flynn

KEYWORDS. Practice applications, direct service, policy, planning, administration, mastery of substantive content, literacy, reward systems, control of technology, computer-assisted systems, mainframes vs. microcomputers, and system control

SUMMARY. The introduction of computers and information technology into the human services requires that particular attention be paid to a number of issues. These include the need for mastery of substantive content prior to introduction of the technology, the definition of computer literacy appropriate to the field, the relative importance of micro- and mainframe computing for practitioners, creation of an adequate reward system for system development, and proper consideration for the sensitive issue of who controls the technology within human services.

This paper surveys selected issues that must be considered with the introduction of computers and information technology into the human services. Particular attention is given to professional prac-

John P. Flynn is Professor of Social Work at the School of Social Work, Western Michigan University, Kalamazoo, MI 49008. He received his MSW from the University of Michigan and his PhD from the Graduate School of Social Work, University of Denver. He teaches in the area of social welfare policy, planning and administration and is an active developer and user of computer-assisted instruction and simulations for teaching and learning about social welfare policy processes. He recently completed a sabbatical in Madrid, Spain, where he conducted research on the tasks of managers of social services and developed a training plan for such managers.

21

tice in direct services and to policy, planning and administration in human services, as opposed to the organizational maintenance or operational affairs involved in these issues.

Direct services refers to the procedures which provide assessment, treatment or planned change for individuals, families, groups, organizations or communities. Policy is defined as "those principles which give expression to valued ends and provide direction to social welfare action" (Flynn, 1985b, p. 6). Policy refers more to the principles embodied in the desired end states or principles that guide action than to the means for attaining such ends, such as direct services. Planning is defined as "the conscious attempt to solve problems and control the course of future events by foresight, systematic thinking, investigation, and the exercise of value preferences in choosing among alternative lines of action" (Gilbert & Specht, 1977, p. 1). The emphasis on planning, then, is on bringing policy choices to fruition through the development and implementation of means, rather than ends. Policy focuses on goals or end states; planning focuses on procedures or the means of attaining goals and objectives. Gates refers to this relationship as the "chain of means and ends" (Gates, 1980, p. 7). Administration is the implementation of policy and plans, as well as the creative orchestration of resources that generates and regenerates new policy and planning opportunities. In reality, the provision of direct services, policy, planning and administration are inextricably interwoven. Each activity is part of the chain in the development, delivery and maintenance of human services.

This discussion explores selected issues involved in seizing opportunities for the application of computer and information technology for the improvement of human services. Some of these applications, such as management information systems, data manipulation in research and evaluation, and program budgeting and fiscal management, are well known. Those applications to human services are more or less similar in their nature to general applications of the technology and need not be discussed in detail here. However, some issues in these applications are worth noting before moving on.

One issue to be mentioned in passing concerns the central importance of maintaining security regarding confidentiality and privacy in computerized management information systems. In human services, confidentiality and privacy have clinical as well as legal ramifications. The protection of human subjects in research and evaluation projects, as it pertains to computer usage or otherwise, is another matter of particular concern in the human service environment. The storage and retrieval of research and evaluation data, particularly as it relates to sensitive clinical information, place citizens at risk if adequate procedures are not ensured. Yet another issue is the importance of the design and use of accounting systems that reflect the unique nature of human service agencies funded and sponsored by a variety of sources and accountable to a variety of monitors. General purpose accounting systems for the profit or business sectors are not designed or suited for this special tracking of revenues and expenditures across funding sources. Special adaptations of computer software are often needed for applications to human service agencies.

The issues engendered by less common or less obvious applications of computer and information technology will be discussed below. Uses such as policy analysis modeling and projection, project planning, networking of various kinds, decision support systems, and computer assisted instruction for training and staff development are perhaps less obvious or more uncommon but emerging applications within the field.

ISSUES IN APPLICATION

Technology introduces or generates a number of issues when merged with professional autonomy, art and science. Not the least of these is the problem of establishing "computer literacy," already noted by Reinoehl and Hanna (1990). LaMendola (1985) has also enumerated a number of the salient issues generally related to these technological applications to the human services. The issues discussed in this paper focus more specifically on: (1) the need for mastery of substantive content as a prerequisite for introducing computer applications, (2) the extent to which the professional person needs to develop "computer literacy," (3) the relative importance of micro- or mainframe computing systems for the human service practitioner, (4) the reward system for those who invest their resources in bringing this technology to the human services, and (5) the question of who shall control the nature and degree of influence of this technology over the field.

Mastery of Substantive Content

The main or central issue lies in the need for professionals to master the substantive content of their practice prior to any attempt at computer application. This view is consistent with the approach taken by Reinoehl and Hanna (1988) in their pursuit of a definition of "computer literacy." In fact, they view literacy as an interrelationship between ability for computer applications and abilities in practice in human services.

As with any intrusion of technology to professional practice, it is essential that the practitioner first have a thorough familiarity with the substantive knowledge, information and skills of the field within which a new technology is introduced. The potential problem is perhaps most evident in a review of the research literature. As Cowger (1984) has appropriately called to our attention, violation of this principle is illustrated in professional journal articles wherein data are analyzed with the use of canned statistical programs without regard to the propriety of a particular statistical application. In many instances, perhaps the attraction of the number crunching capabilities of the computer has led to indiscriminant use of the hardware and software. Part of that problem may be due to a lack of adequate preparation in selection of appropriate statistical techniques. However, much is likely due to use of the computer simply because "it is there." The result is an inappropriate substantive application.

A common saying is: "If you want to really mess up the procedure, use a computer to do it!" or "If you think this is bad, you should see it when we use the computer!" Both of these comments cleverly mask the reality that it is not the computer, with a mind of its own so to speak, but the *person* or *system* that inappropriately confounds the application. In this instance, the machine takes the brunt of the blame. It is the manager of the machinery who is really to blame; the machine-blaming phenomenon is, perhaps, only a result of the behavior of applying technology before mastering the content that the technology was supposed to serve.

The introduction of any technology or tool into a process or procedure requires that the goals and objectives of the intervention are, a priori, very clear. In this day of burgeoning uses of computer technology, we are often enticed by the availability of all kinds of "friendly" programs, by our enthusiasm for "efficiency" (which, of course, may or may not be afforded by a computer application), and sometimes even a selfish need to play with our new toys. But computers (or any electronic or mechanical machinery, for that matter) cannot set goals and objectives or order priorities. Machinery can only manipulate the substantive information provided by humans and, at times, only fulfill the logical plan given in a set of instructions. The use of machinery to perform functions assigned solely to humans is a misuse of both human and non-human resources. It is when the professional practitioner has mastery over his or her substantive content that the technology can provide an appropriate supplement to practice.

The use of computerized diagnostic and assessment programs, such as self-administered intake procedures or personality profiles obtained on a computer, are valuable aids to clinical treatment. So, too, are computer-assisted project management systems, such as PERT, flow-charting and GANTT charting. However, the use of these applications without a clear understanding of their strengths and limitations is irresponsible. The products of computer output are meaningless, perhaps even dangerous, if the practitioner is not firmly grounded in the subject matter for which the technology is employed in the service or problem-solving.

The use of nonhuman resources demands human control and mastery of substantive content. Human resources must be served, not controlled, by nonhuman devices. Professionals in human services have an ethical responsibility to carefully examine the propriety of a computer application for a particular task prior to the decision to employ the technology.

Computer Literacy

Given the presumption that the use of technology first requires mastery of one's substantive content or field of practice, the next issue is generated by questions of how one is equipped to select the application and of how computer literacy will be defined. As

Reinoehl and Hanna have helped conceptualize the problem, the issues of mastery in practice and computer application are really intricately interrelated. "Computer literacy" is dependent upon "practice literacy."

The content and criteria for determining literacy and proficiency are yet to be established, though the matrix developed by Reinoehl and Hanna (1988) suggests a number of examples of levels of ability in each area. Both computer ability and professional practice ability move through a continuum from beginning awareness, to a level of proficiency in application or practice, and on to the level of the ability for creative development.

A central issue that divides many in determining what constitutes "computer literacy" or "competency" is whether or not a professional computer user needs to master at least one programming language. The argument in favor of programming language "literacy" suggests that the ability to understand the logic of systematically issuing a set of executable commands to the machinery enables a more complete understanding of the technology. Presumably, this mastery will lead to more effective and appropriate use. Others would say that programming ability is not necessary in order to become "computer literate." This opposing argument holds that, since there are numerous "user friendly" application programs available, programming in source language or assembly language is not necessary. Examples are found in the proliferation of spreadsheets and data base management systems; more recently, expert systems for querying are more and more based upon the principle of maintaining high level, near-human language commands. This logic suggests that a preoccupation with the essentials of source programming language diverts the user from a proper focus upon the substantive content of the problem or task. Consequently, the issues of mastery of substantive content and the primacy of computer literacy become interrelated. Furthermore, potential efficiencies to be gained in the use of the technology are often lost in time-consuming software program development.

Clearly mastery in the practice area does not require mastery in programming in assembly languages or PASCAL or C or the like. Insistence upon such skill would be the equivalent of requiring all social researchers to be able to illustrate the mathematical derivation of all statistical formulas employed in social research, as if all social scientists must also function at the level of terminal-degreed statisticians. However, this is not to deny the fact that proficiency in programming at any level could not be said to be the creative development level of competence and that functioning at that level should be welcomed and encouraged in those who are so inclined.

Many efficiencies in computer programming are obtained by the availability of higher levels of machine instruction, such as macros and authoring languages. Macros provide for a series of instructions in the use of canned programs; authoring languages also allow for calling in frequently used routines in preparing computer-assisted instruction. The question has to be asked whether these levels of computer "programming" do not, in themselves, constitute computer literacy in the context of professional practice since the user is able to manipulate the machinery by these sophisticated and "friendly" means of ordering a series of instructions (i.e., of "programming").

This issue of literacy requirements must be resolved by human service professionals themselves if proper standards are to be developed for the preparation of human services staff. When the standards for that literacy are established, whether formally or informally, professionals will need training and guidance. Human service professionals will either have to possess their own independence through competence in both areas or will need to recognize the need for direction by others outside of the field. Human service professionals will need to determine for themselves the proper conditions for seeking and selecting outside assistance.

A Mainframe vs. Microcomputer Emphasis

The next issue would appear, on the surface, as being more technical in nature since it involves making choices between hardware, i.e., between mainframe or microcomputer systems development. However, the issue is beyond mere hardware selection and goes to the heart of how and why computer and information *systems* are to serve the clientele of human services in the first place.

As occurred in other fields, the computer was first introduced in the human services as a mainframe machine, primarily for storage of large databases, in creating management information systems, or in using financial packages for inventory control or accounting systems. Initially, computing was synonymous with mainframe computing on large machines, the process of which was controlled by a priesthood who tended the service in strange languages. More recently, computing for many has become synonymous with microcomputing. Given increased power, availability, reduced size and cost, and increased user sophistication, this turn of events is perhaps fortuitous and appropriate. However, it is as if "camps" have evolved, creating large gaps in awareness of differential mainframe and micro-computing applications. Some have lost, at least temporarily, a vision of computing *systems* with a range of software and hardware characteristics, from small to large machines and programs. New developments in the area of networking, time-sharing, and stand-alone capabilities have since come along.

There is no longer a clear division between the mainframe- and micro-based computing systems. This division is, of course, unnecessary today and was, developmentally speaking, only a temporary indicator of the state of technological application to the human services. Nevertheless, human service professionals must recognize what appears to be a dysfunctional chauvinism or naive fadism found in making unnecessary choices of one type of a system over another. To be sure, micro-based systems are more available and affordable to the majority of human service professional users. But current availability and affordability should not be the criteria employed in planning for the future. Useful applications for clinical practice and policy, planning and administration are to be found in the range of computer system capabilities in which mainframe and microcomputing are each exploited for their maximum potential. A good example of the mix of both mainframe and microcomputing (and minicomputing) hardware is found in the growth of local area networks, bulletin board systems, and electronic mail. This development should not be overlooked.

For the human service practitioner, this provides a challenge to the myopic view of either categorical mainframe or solely microcomputing literacy. In one area, we can anticipate a shift from a reliance upon large mainframe computer systems when large data base management systems are involved. Given the increased miniaturization, power, and affordability of hard discs and mass storage devices for microcomputers, the reliance on mainframes for those applications are disappearing. When the data bases need not be accessed or updated by a large number of users on demand, microcomputing would appear to be in order. On the other hand, given the nightmares involved in evaluating and storing user performance on computer-assisted instruction systems for staff development and training, it is difficult to see when micro-based systems will ever be appropriate for large staff development and training programs. The logistics of updating lessons on floppy discs distributed over a wide geographic area is, in itself, a task for large, centralized computing and information systems. Surely large electronic mail systems, electronic bulletin boards and other forms of networking illustrate the increasing interdependence between *systems* involving *both* mainframe- and micro-based computing capacity.

The Reward for Investment

Except for the management and fiscal information system applications noted above, as well as the uses in research and statistical analysis, computers are relatively new to the human services. Given this newness, the initial investment in learning and applying the technology has fallen, perhaps even voluntarily or without any planning, to a relatively few human service professionals. There are examples in the literature of applications in developing decision support systems (Jaffe, 1979; Gripton, 1980; Schoech & Schkade, 1980; Boyd et al., 1981) or computer-assisted instruction (Flynn, M., 1977; Luse, 1980; Flynn, 1985a, 1987; Flynn & Kuczeruk, 1984) which require enormous investments of time and energy.

However, the level of effort needed to produce the new materials and procedures required to obtain mastery and control of the technology have not generally been appropriately acknowledged by professional performance evaluation systems. This is largely due to the fact that it is difficult to assign value to a new technology. The personal costs incurred in the use of a strange new technology are often not appreciated or adequately evaluated. At worst, those who experiment with new technological applications are often seen by other professionals as "nerds" or people who inappropriately apply machinery to human systems. At best, other professional colleagues may have a simplistic and overly respectful understanding of what computers involve and expect the developer to simply "push the right button" in order to magically produce fantastic technical results.

As compared to traditional means of professional recognition, such as the conduct of research, consultation, community participation and service, publication, and the like, the role of developing computer applications has not been adequately built into recognition or compensation schemes for professional status and advancement. Until the reward system is adjusted to appropriately acknowledge computer application efforts, the technology will be underutilized or inappropriately applied. Incentives for development and proper exploitation of this resource will be lacking.

The Maintenance of System Control

As incentives and rewards for computer system development emerge, and as statuses are assigned to those who have been "anointed to the priesthood," the question remains as to who will stand in control of technology's application. Part of the answer depends upon how the question of computer literacy, discussed above, is resolved.

Proponents of one position on literacy would suggest that a thorough familiarity with software and hardware functioning by the professional user is essential if the user is to maintain proper control over the technology's usage. Given familiarity with the basics of the machine's functioning, one is presumed to be able to take command not only of the machine but also the systems that relate to the technology's use. Proponents of the other position would hold that resources and energy allocated to obtain such mastery is unnecessarily expended. Instead, those who have the requisite competencies for applications could properly serve under the direction of human service professionals with selected training in the use of computer and information technology. Clinicians, policy makers, planners and administrators can hire, consult with, or obtain guidance from computer technicians or computer scientists. What the field must strive for, whether obtained by consultation or independent practice, is achievement of Reinhoehl and Hanna's competencies included in the upper right-hand quadrant of their matrix of computer and practice abilities. The goals of competence should be paramount. We need to argue less about the means and focus more on the goals of merging these areas of practice and application.

CONCLUSION

Computer applications in the human services raise questions about: (1) the substantive goal, objective or issue for which the computer is selected as a problem-solving tool, (2) the demands to be placed upon the practitioner for the essential and appropriate level of computer literacy to perform the task, (3) the appropriate level and scale of hardware and software for the job or task to be completed, (4) sufficient professional incentives, satisfaction and rewards for those who produce the applications, in comparison to other available alternatives for professional growth and organizational development, and (5) the resolution of the issue of who shall control the computing and information systems applied to human services.

Clearly, we have much work to do to confront these issues. In the area of mastery of substantive content, we need to find ways to assure ourselves that we are, in fact, ready to apply the technology to a given task or problem. We need to develop a litmus test, so to speak, to determine when the technological application is ready, based upon our thorough understanding of the substantive nature and content of the matter at hand. This means we need to also develop skill in testing and identifying the boundaries of our own knowledge — of both the substantive content within which we are practicing and the use of computer and information technology.

As to computer literacy, we will need to expand our awareness of the range and variety of existing hardware and software available so that we do not foolishly and unknowingly commit ourselves and our resources to inappropriate systems. Our charge will constantly be that of testing the "goodness of fit" between the technological application and the requirements of the substantive issues. This will push us to obtaining ever higher orders of specificity in what we need and demand of the technology. Given that goal achieved, we will need to dedicate ourselves to mastery of what is available.

Our skills in interpersonal and interorganizational networking will be put to the test as we realize the merger of both computer and information technologies with the human services. As we achieve our goals in that area, it will be essential that we take and maintain control of these new advances that must not only serve our own purposes but, ultimately, the clients and consumers of human services.

In short, we have many expectations. But are the expectations any more revolutionary than the issues generated by the introduction of other tools, such as the pencil and paper, the telephone, or the photocopier into human service delivery systems? Perhaps what is at issue here is our ability to give direction and to take control of this technology's impact upon the human services.

REFERENCES

Boyd, L. Jr., Pruger, R., Chase, M. D., Clark, M. & Miller, L. S. (1981). A decision support system to increase equity. *Administration in Social Work*, 5(3/4), 83-96.

Cowger, C. D. (1984). Statistical significance tests: Scientific ritualism or scientific method? *Social Service Review*, 8(3), 358-372.

Flynn, J. P. (1985a). MERGE: Computer simulations of social policy process. *Computers in Human Services*, 1(2), 33-45.

Flynn, J. P. (1985b). *Social agency policy: Analysis and presentation for community practice*. Chicago, IL: Nelson-Hall Publishers.

Flynn, J. P. (1987). Simulating policy processes through electronic mail. *Computers in Human Services*, 2(1/2):13-26.

Flynn, J. P. & Kuczeruk, T. (1984). Computer-assisted instruction for the private practitioner. In M. D. Schwartz, (Ed.), *Using computers in clinical practice*. (pp. 395-416). New York: The Haworth Press.

Flynn, M. L. (1977). Computer-based instruction in social policy: A one-year trial. *Journal of Education for Social Work*, 13(1), 52-59.

Gates, B. L. (1980). *Social program administration: The implementation of social policy*, Englewood Cliffs, NJ: Prentice-Hall, Inc.

Gilbert, N. & Specht, H. (1977). *Planning for social welfare: Issues, models and tasks*. Englewood Cliffs, NJ: Prentice-Hall, Inc.

Gripton, J. (March, 1980). Applications of systems analysis and computer simulation to the administration of social welfare services. Paper presented at the meeting of the Council on Social Work Education, Los Angeles, CA.

Jaffe, E. D. (1979). Computers in child placement planning. *Social Work*, 24(5), 380-385.

LaMendola, W. F. (1985). The future of human service information technology: An essay on the number 42. *Computers in Human Services*, 1(1), 35-49.

Luse, F. D. (1980). Use of computer simulation in social welfare management. *Administration in Social Work*, *4*, 13-22.

Reinhoehl, R. & Hanna, T. (1990). Defining computer literacy. *Computers in Human Services*, this volume.

Schoech, D. & Schkade, L. L. (1980). Computers helping caseworkers: Decision support systems. *Child Welfare*, Nov. 566-575.

SECTION II:
OFF-THE-SHELF SOFTWARE
AND ITS UTILITY IN HUMAN SERVICES

Introduction

During the last few years in-house computers have become the rule rather than the exception in the world of human services. Administrators and boards have agreed on the importance of the new machines as management tools, and there has been some exploration of direct computer use by staff and clients. Thus the computer has become a necessity for agencies and organizations which wish to keep a competitive edge and for directors who realize that computers can help manage the ever greater quantities of information necessary for daily operations.

What is not so evident is whether or not the hardware is being utilized effectively. Up until the early 1980s, the computer was still primarily a management-oriented number cruncher. State-level social service agencies, for example, maintain sophisticated management information systems that allow for client career tracking, cost analyses, and personnel management databases. In the past, such large agencies (and some smaller ones) also maintained stand alone computers that had a dedicated use, such as word processing or client billing.

In other cases, smaller agencies either used a timesharing approach or maintained their own small computer for accounting purposes or for specialized tasks, such as client record maintenance, client assessment or related information capturing functions. Additionally, some few agencies came to utilize the search and extract capabilities of the growing number of online databases such as ERIC or Psych Abstracts. Such uses were appropriate to the computer technology available at the time and remain appropriate today.

In the meantime, however, both hardware and software have gone through several surges of development, and our experiences have shown that human service organizations (like many other organizations) have been slow in taking full advantage of these developments. Without dwelling on the reasons for this situation we assert that it should be possible, in fact expected, that agencies exploit these new resources. It is to this expectation that we dedicate this section, and encourage the reader to contribute to the creative use of readily available off-the-shelf applications in solving human service problems.

Computer Assisted Life Review

Richard Reinoehl
Helen Brown
Linda D. Iroff

KEYWORDS. Aging, life review, developmental stages, life crises, ego-integrity, idea precessors, outliners, computers, direct service

SUMMARY. A positive life review process is crucial to the resolution of the last of Ericson's developmental life crises, ego-integrity vs. despair. This paper describes and discusses: (1) the importance of the life review process and life review therapy; (2) the nature of idea processors, a type of computer software; and (3) ways that idea processors can be useful in facilitating a therapeutic life review process for elderly individuals.

INTRODUCTION

Microcomputers have become common place in human service organizations with a major focus on programs for administrative uses: electronic spreadsheets, word processors, and data management programs (Doucette, 1985). Direct client/computer contact

---

Richard Reinoehl is Director of the Human Development Consortium, Inc., a computer consulting group working with human service organizations and educational institutions, 24 Uptown Village, Ithaca, NY 14850. He is a past faculty of the Social Work Program, University of Wisconsin, Superior.

Helen Brown is employed by the American Association of Retired Person's Andrus Foundation to review proposals and make funding recommendations. She is a past faculty in the Human Services Program, College of Human Ecology, Cornell University, Ithaca, NY 14853.

Linda D. Iroff is a computer support specialist for the College of Arts and Sciences, Cornell University, Ithaca, NY 14853.

(regardless of computer type or size) is less usual, and in clinical practice has primarily dealt with assessment rather than treatment. Currently, the use of computers to assist the elderly has focused on its use as a prosthesis for the disabled and as a recreational device to fill leisure time and to prevent decline in reaction time (McGuire, 1986). Thus, the direct use of computers to enhance the quality of clients' lives is still a relatively unexplored area, although possibly one of the richest in terms of using the computer as a resource.

Since the development of computer software is an expensive and time consuming process, software has usually been targeted for the business community. With the exception of medical and psychological treatment, human services are not often seen as lucrative enough for software companies to specifically target software; and although grant money is sometimes available, human service organizations usually do not have the time, expertise or money to write much software for themselves.

A consequence of this situation is the dearth of software for direct service involving client/computer interaction, which is especially true in the area of aging. Although this is frustrating for the direct service practitioner, a solution is to use existing software in creative ways. One such application uses idea processors or outliners, as a way for the elderly to work through the life review process. Idea processors are easy to use, and require no programming knowledge. Thus, individuals can create and implement products that respond to local conditions, i.e., significant historical community events and local cultural and ethnic influences within the population.

This paper will: (1) describe and discuss the importance of the life review process, (2) explain idea processors, and (3) suggest ways that these two bodies of knowledge can be integrated for use by activity directors in institutions. Of course, this process is also useful for others who work with the elderly and wish to aid their clients (or family) in the life review process.

DEVELOPMENT AND LIFE REVIEW

The elderly are constantly writing and rewriting the scenarios of their lives (Butler, 1975), and developmentalists argue that this facilitates dealing with a major developmental task of old age: resolution of the crises of ego-integrity vs. despair. Havigursts (1973) proposes that distinct psycho-social tasks associated with each stage of life must be mastered for an individual to enjoy a sense of satisfaction and success at any particular stage. Fenkel-Brunswik (1963) defined the task of old age as that of integration and acceptance of one's whole life history. Ericson (1968) characterized the developmental stage of late life crises of ego-integrity vs. despair as the time to find "order and meaning." While integration leads to a state of integration, despair is the result of the failure to integrate.

Old age inaugurates the life review process, a universal occurrence, by stimulating the realization of approaching dissolution and death (Butler, ibid.). Life review is characterized by the progressive return to consciousness of past experiences, in particular the resurgence of unresolved conflicts which in late life can be surveyed and re-integrated. Although the review is more commonly known as reminiscence, it includes, but is not limited to reminiscence. The old are not only taking stock of themselves as they review their lives, they are thinking and feeling through what they will do with the time that is left and considering whatever emotional and material legacies they may have to give to others. Fallot (1980) pointed out that life review is not a response to motivation to live in the past; but rather, a normal process of identity consolidation and personality integration.

Formalized life review is an organized process to facilitate the reviewing of one's life in order to help the individual to reflect on and to understand the importance or meaning of experiences for the past, and their meaning for the present and future. There is evidence that resolution of the ego integrity-despair issue is facilitated through recollecting contributions made, rewards received, accomplishments and failures. Successful integration of unresolved conflicts and fears can give more significance and meaning to an individual's life and help prepare him for death, mitigating his fears.

Butler (ibid.) noted that reminiscence of the old has often been devalued; and is felt to bespeak of aimless wandering of the mind or living in the past. However, reminiscence is seen in the great memoirs composed in old age which provide fascinating accounts of history which otherwise would not exist. Several universities, recognizing the historical value of memoirs, have "Oral History Collection" programs to obtain and preserve memories of individuals from all walks of life.

Life Review Therapy

Life review therapy refers to various means that are used to facilitate a positive life review process. These can include the taking of extensive autobiographies from older persons, developing genealogies, creating scrapbooks of an individual's history, etc., which invoke crucial memories, responses, and understanding of a person's life work. Among the positive outcomes of these activities include the expiation of guilt, exorcism of problematic childhood identifications, the transmission of knowledge and values to those who follow and the renewal of ideas of citizenship (Butler & Lewis, 1974). Several special characteristics of the aged make clear the value of the life review in regard to these outcomes.

First, as older persons are sometimes chased by feelings of guilt, they attempt to resurrect and come to terms with regretted past acts of commission and of omission. Secondly, older persons have nostalgic memorial attachment to familiar objects, e.g., home, pets, heirlooms, keepsakes, photo albums, scrapbooks, old letters. These familiar objects provide a sense of continuity, comfort, security and satisfaction. Viewing and reflecting on these can jog the mind and encourage memories of the immediate and distant past. Third, the elderly need opportunities to appraise, extract, and pass on that which they feel is worthy knowledge to younger generations to achieve a sense of continuity. Finally, older persons have the need to feel a sense of legacy. Thus, they have a profound need to leave something behind when they die. Although some may have works of art or treasured family possessions, for others this legacy consists of the memories of their contribution in terms of their life, its struggles and triumphs (Butler & Lewis, ibid).

Butler and Lewis also state that, ". . . life review therapy can be conducted in a variety of settings from senior centers to nursing homes. Even relatively untrained persons can function as therapists by becoming 'listeners' as older persons recount their lives." However, to listen is often time consuming, with little apparent benefit to the listener. (The listener could be learning, but the need for an elderly person to review and re-review episodes would become boring—and from an organizational view would not be cost-effective.) Fortunately, computer assisted life review therapy utilizing idea processors offers a solution to this problem.

IDEA PROCESSING

Idea processors (also called outline or thought processors) provide a means for organizing and reorganizing thoughts, both textually and pictorially. They allow the user to create outlines and freely reorganize headings, subheadings, text, and graphics. Other features include the ability to attach text or graphics to a heading, sort through and prioritize lists, expand or contact the outline to view any level of headings (e.g., major headings or specified subheadings), and link the material to a word processor.

For example, a user can make a list of headings on a specific topic. As new ideas are thought of, they can be placed on the outline as new headings or subheadings. The order, or chronology, of headings can be changed. Subheadings can be moved to higher (more important) levels, or relegated to sub, subheading status as needed. Thus the outline can be continually expanded and revised as conception of the material becomes more integrated.

There are several idea processors that are commercially available from a variety of vendors with a price range of power, flexibility, ease of use and price. Programs are available for most computers including the Macintosh, Apple II, and IBM PC and compatibles. In addition, many word processing programs now include outlining features of this nature. Some of these programs are low in cost and very easy to use.

INTEGRATION

The way that an idea processor can be used to facilitate the life review process can be seen from two primary views, i.e., the developer and the user. In the first case, two tasks must be considered, (1) stimulating the memory of the aging individual, and (2) placing the review process into a positive, therapeutic context. The completion of these tasks would result in two outlines (in two separate files), one historical and the other developmental, which each individual user could use to begin his or her own life history.

The Developer's View

Stimulating the memory of a user can be accomplished by incorporating past local, national, and international events into an idea processing file. This can include photographs, newspaper headlines and stories of key events and people. Libraries and newspaper offices have a wealth of historic information usable for such purposes. Text can be typed or scanned into a computer and photographs can be digitized and incorporated at a low cost using commonly available technology (although quality can vary considerably among differing digitizers). Using some computers' ability to provide a variety of on-screen fonts, font sizes, and graphics and text mixing, facsimiles of actual newspaper stories could even be created and stored.

Primary headings, in order of occurrence, can speak to eras that encompass several, or even many years. Some examples are: World War I, the Roaring Twenties, the Great Depression, World War II, etc. Subheadings would include major events that were involved in that era, e.g., the bombing of Pearl Harbor would be one of several major events of World War II. Dates would be included, of course. Additional sub, subheadings, et cetera, can fill-in with the chronology of lesser events that sequentially occurred. Text and graphics that describe an era or event would be included under each heading and subheading.

This event oriented approach seems reasonable, as it is events that create impacts on individuals, not the year or date itself. However, events impact differently on individuals and a developer will find his or her self making value judgements regarding the importance of an event. For instance, how much of an event was Elvis Presley's appearance on the Ed Sullivan Show? How does this compare with the election of John Kennedy over Richard Nixon, the Cardinals winning the World Series, or Mary Pickford's marriage to Douglas Fairbanks? Since an individual will place a different value on an event, or category of events (such as politics or sports) than their neighbor, how does a developer decide on a specific value structure when creating a hierarchical structure of events?

One answer would be to make several historical outlines, each with a particular class of events having a higher value in the hierarchical structure. Duplicating an outline and then altering the structure and other re-placement of events is an easy task with an idea processor and is within the realm of practical consideration. However, a better answer is for a developer to make his or her best judgement based on the extent of the general social impact of the event, and then *let the user restructure the outline into the form best representing their values and life experiences.*

The second task, creating a therapeutic context, would involve providing textual and graphic images that would enhance an individuals understanding of interpersonal processes, human development and emotional growth. There are an ample number of journals and books which provide information on human development from birth to very old age. Some of these texts not only look at issues of individual development at differing ages, but also explore social interrelationships from a developmental view.

Knowledge about stages of development can be helpful for elderly in terms of understanding certain aspects of their past and current life, and providing a context for their own integration of life experiences. Other information of a therapeutic nature is also generally available and can be used. For instance, knowledge of family dynamics can be useful in this regard; one example could involve why and how family scapegoats emerge. This type of knowledge can help an individual place old actions and feelings into a context that aids in an understanding that resolves an old emotional conflict.

There are several ways to approach the use of an idea processor for facilitating life review. One is to use a sequential approach regarding development. That is, topic headings would start with birth and move through early childhood with a stage by stage progression toward old age. Subheadings for each age would involve topics relevant to activities and interests of that age. Narrative text and relevant graphics would accompany each outline topic.

Besides these two tasks, another concern for a developer is the difficulty of the computer system and the training time involved for a novice computer user. Training time will vary from person to person and is beyond the control of a developer. However, the choice of which computer system to use is within a developer's domain, and a computer which uses a graphic user interface (such as the Macintosh) would provide a friendly and easy-to-use system. Thus, training time can be kept to a minimum and a novice user can immediately begin their computer assisted life review.

The User's View

Control of this carefully constructed presentation of information passes to the user after their first orientation to the system. The user's first choice is to decide whether to use the history file, the developmental file, the word processing program, or directly access the idea processor. The latter two choices would allow the user to proceed with creating their own life review before referring to what the developer has prepared. This choice would present itself as icons (see Figure I)* and the user would use a mouse to point to (and double-clicking the mouse button to "open," or access) their preference.

Assuming a desire to explore one of the developer's files, the user might open the Life Development file. What would next appear on the screen would be the primary headings of the stages of life development as shown in Figure II. Supposing an interest in one particular stage, the user could open the narrative and graphic images which provide information on typical aspects of this stage. Then he or she could open any or all of the subheadings (and their narrative/graphics) that would allow a more specific exploration of a topic.

Figure III shows how a computer screen could look after a narrative and subheadings under "Adolescence" were opened. Other levels of subheadings could be opened and explored, and sub, subheadings also could be opened for narratives and graphics which would deal with those aspects of development.

Behaviorally, a specific heading or subheading would be opened by double clicking the mouse in the circle associated with the topic.

---

*All figures use a facsimile of a Macintosh screen; menus, scroll bars, and trash and disk icons are not shown. Generic names, graphics and processes are used to represent application programs.

The Screen After Inserting Disk

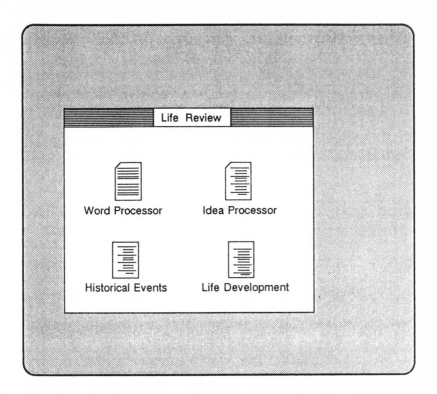

Figure I

Double clicking on the topic itself would open the topic narrative, and topics would be re-located by clicking dragging them to their new location. Thus the user would need only a small repertoire of activities in order to explore and manipulate this environment.

Another choice exists for the user who now wishes to begin recording their own life story. They can either create their own life review file, or begin modifying the developmental history file into their life story. As an example, under the topic "Adolescence," subtopic "Family," a user could begin typing, "When I was thir-

The Initial Headings For Stages of Life

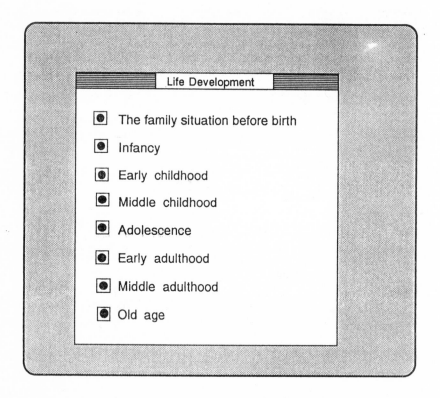

The family situation before birth

Infancy

Early childhood

Middle childhood

Adolescence

Early adulthood

Middle adulthood

Old age

Life Development

Figure II

teen, the twins were born and Mom had her breakdown — and gave up trying to raise her five children. As the oldest I had to take over running the household including taking care of Mom. I was scared at first, but eventually became good at it. I did not know it at the time, but this has effected how I have lived the rest of my life. When I think about it now, I . . ."

Once this reminiscence is completed, the user can keep it under that subheading, or change the subheading from "Adolescence —

Opening The Next Level of Specificity

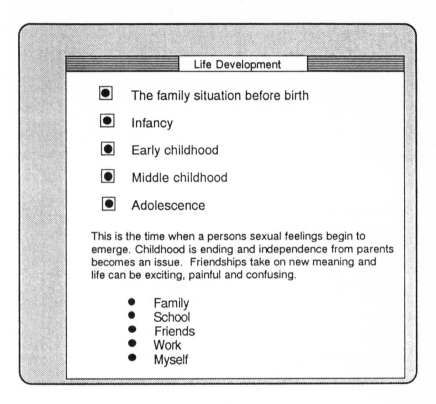

Life Development

☉ The family situation before birth

☉ Infancy

☉ Early childhood

☉ Middle childhood

☉ Adolescence

This is the time when a persons sexual feelings begin to emerge. Childhood is ending and independence from parents becomes an issue. Friendships take on new meaning and life can be exciting, painful and confusing.

- Family
- School
- Friends
- Work
- Myself

Figure III

Family'' to "Mom's breakdown," and move it to the position of a major heading due to its importance of having strongly effected the development of the individual's life. As this person continues her reminiscence and begins to integrate and accept various aspects of her life history, she could change her mind about the importance of "Mom's breakdown" and again alter the structure or content of her life review file. At anytime a copy of a life review file can be transferred into a regular word processing file or even a desktop publishing program; portions could also be copied and incorporated into letters and sent to family or friends. Thus, what was initially the product of the developer gradually becomes the life story of an individual user.

CONCLUSION

From the preceding, one can see how commercially available software can be innovatively applied to help solve a human services problem. It is the belief of the authors that there currently exists a broad range of relatively inexpensive, commonly available computer programs that, although not originally designed for human services, can become quite useful when applied in a creative manner.

In this particular case, we have shown how idea processors, combined with word processors and graphics programs, could be beneficial in facilitating the life review process — possibly the most important element in a successful culmination of an individual's life. One aspect of the use of idea processors for this task is that a local developer can create such a system without knowledge of how to use a programming language, and can easily adapt their product to local events and cultures.

In use of such an application, individual users would begin with a structure of historic and psycho-social information created by a human services professional. From this, the users can choose — and modify — the information they wish to utilize in their own life story. Thus the control over the computer-assisted life review process passes to the users with their first introduction to the system; it is theirs to arrange and rearrange according to their interpretation — as each finds new order and meaning in life

BIBLIOGRAPHY

Butler, R. N. (1975). Successful aging and the role of the life review. In Zaris, S. H. (Ed) *Readings in Aging and Death*. New York: Harper & Row.

Butler, R. N. & Lewis, M. I. (1977). *Aging and mental health: Positive psychosocial approaches (Second Edition)*. St. Louis: Mosby.

Doucette, Jr., J. A. (1985). *A Directory of Microcomputer Software in the Human Services*. Maine, Portland: Computer Consulting and Programming Associates.

Fallot, R. D. (1980). The impact on mood of verbal reminiscing in later adulthood. *International Journal of Aging and Human Development, 10,* 385-400.

Frenkel-Brunswik, E. (1963). Adjustment and reorientation in the course of the life span. In Kuhler, R. G. & Thompsen, G. G. (Eds) *Psychological Studies of Human Development (Second Edition)*. New York: Appleton-Century-Crofts.

Havighurst, R. J. (1973). History of developmental psychology: Socialization and personality development through the life span. In Bates, P. B. & Schaie, K. W. (Eds) *Lifespan Development Psychology: Personality and Socialization*. New York: Academic Press.

McGuire, F. A. (Editor) (1986). *Computer Technology and the Aged: Implications and Activities for Activity Programs*. New York: The Haworth Press.

Spreadsheet Analysis in Human Services

Fred V. Janzen
Robert E. Lewis

KEYWORDS. Computers, spreadsheets, social service, human service, clinical measurement, program monitoring, computer simulations, automated eligibility, form development

SUMMARY. Computerized spreadsheets were developed to support accounting functions, but these programs have come to have much broader applications. This chapter introduces spreadsheet analysis, briefly explains key concepts used in creating spreadsheets, and finally gives examples from direct practice and human service administration. While spreadsheets can be used for any task that requires manipulation of numbers or use of a calculator, they are most useful in producing charts and tables and for modeling problems requiring "what if" projections.

This chapter introduces spreadsheet analysis and briefly explains key concepts used in creating spreadsheets. Examples of several useful spreadsheet applications in human services are depicted. First, some applications of spreadsheet programs in direct practice settings are shown. These examples demonstrate graphic display

Fred V. Janzen, BS, MSW, PhD, is Associate Professor, Graduate School of Social Work, University of Utah. His areas of interest include: social use of computer technology, information utilization, conducting assessment surveys, contract and program monitoring, program evaluation research, and applied social statistics. He has taught computer technology to social work students for the past 15 years.

Robert E. Lewis, BS, MS, MSW, is a doctoral candidate, Graduate School of Social Work, University of Utah. He is also Research Consultant, Utah Division of Family Services. His areas of interest include: child welfare and family treatment, clinical practice research, program evaluation, management information utilization, social service information systems, and information systems planning.

51

and trend analysis of client functioning measures. Next, an approach to the development and tracking of program performance indicators is provided. A third example shows the use of the spreadsheet capability to model alternatives for program decision-making. The final example demonstrates the creation of an automated service application form in a spreadsheet environment.

Implementing accountability within any human service agency often involves the manipulation and reporting of information typically in the form of numbers and tables. In the not too distant past, large main-frame computers helped to manage data manipulation and analysis. Today, computer use is rapidly decentralizing from desk-size machines in a faraway air-conditioned room to desk-top office microcomputers an arm's length away. At the same time, data-analysis programs that run on these personal computers have become cheaper yet more powerful in their capabilities as well as easier to use by people unfamiliar with computer technology.

Agency personnel who prepare and update financial and statistical records or are concerned with "what-if" questions will want to use one of the newer "spreadsheet" programs. The use of menus and preprogrammed function keys make these electronic spreadsheet programs relatively easy to learn and utilize. Once familiar with the electronic spreadsheet's powerful analytic capabilities and applications, staff are able to produce complex and routine reports more quickly and accurately.

The term *spreadsheet* comes from the ledger sheets accountants use to "spread" rows and columns of numbers out so their relationships can be visually grasped. A computer spreadsheet program is like the accountant's ledger except it is much larger, faster, very accurate and powerful. One major advantage of computer spreadsheets is that if one or several numbers are in error or need to be adjusted, such changes can be easily made without the frustration of having to obliterate large work areas and then re-enter numerous hand calculations. This feature was the motivation that led Dan Bricklin in 1978 to design the first computer spreadsheet to ease his homework, because he was tired of the tedious recalculations required in the financial analysis of case studies in a business course he was taking in the Harvard MBA program. Shortly afterward, *VisiCalc*, the first and very popular spreadsheet package was designed and marketed for the personal computer. Other reliable and equally popular packages being sold today are *SuperCalc*, *Lotus 1-2-3*, *Excel*, *Benchmark Financial Planner*, and *Wingz*. Some of the newer integrated spreadsheet packages have word processing and data-management capabilities that can combine separate but similar spreadsheets, as well as display and print graphics.

An electronic spreadsheet is a time-saving computer software tool useful in organizing information and data into columns and rows. You can make the spreadsheet total, multiply or divide rows and columns of numbers, as well as perform very complex calculations. Mathematical relationships can easily be created between cells of data. The spreadsheet allows you to change any number and see those changes automatically reflected in every part of the spreadsheet related to that number. An electronic spreadsheet can test your creativity in several ways. The latter part of this chapter displays a few ways spreadsheets can be applied to human service agencies.

While spreadsheets can be used for any task that requires manipulation of numbers or use of a calculator, they are most useful in producing charts and tables and for modeling problems requiring "what if" projections. Once a set of mathematical relationships has been built into the spreadsheet, it can be recalculated quickly, depending upon differing assumptions. Agency planners soon find electronic spreadsheets invaluable when managing or forecasting personnel needs, budget changes, and resource reallocations. For instance, "what if" you are required to absorb a five percent budget cut, or "what if" part of the project takes twice as long as anticipated? Using a spreadsheet, an administrator can analyze an array of caseload figures for planning personnel staffing requirements. Spreadsheet analysis allows managers to determine the effect of potential problems and what allowances would be necessary should they occur.

KEY SPREADSHEET CONCEPTS

The workspace of the electronic spreadsheet is divided into several *rows* and *columns* depending on computer memory available. For example, Lotus 1-2-3 and Excel provide hundreds of columns and thousand of rows on each sheet. The columns of the spreadsheet are labeled across the top with letters starting with "A" and extending to the right, say to "BK". The rows are labeled down the left side from "1" through the maximum row allowed.

The intersection of any row and column is designated as a *cell* and is identified by its column and row coordinates, e.g., "A1" or "AH1800." A *range* of cells would be rectangular designation from the beginning cell through the ending cell, such as A7..A10 or AA1..AC20. The *Home* position of the spreadsheet always refers to upper left position of the matrix (i.e., cell "A1") or the beginning of the spreadsheet. A cell can store either of four types of information: numbers or data, labels or text, mathematical equations or formulas, or special spreadsheet functions.

Labels are commonly used for row and column headings. They can be several characters long and can contain any string of characters and numbers. If a label is too long for the width of a cell, it will be displayed across the cells to the right as long as there is no entry in the neighboring cell. Labels are left-justified in the cell, but may be centered or right-justified if desired.

A *function* is a special formula which performs complex calculations on a specified range of cells or data values, such as @SUM-(B1..E1) — to sum the data values found in B1 thru E1 inclusively — or @AVG(F3..F27) — to sum the data values and divide by the number of items to derive an average. Most spreadsheets include arithmetic functions, trigonometric functions, statistical functions, financial functions, selection functions, logical functions, date functions, and database statistical functions. For example, the special function @ERR places "ERR" in the cell if the formula cannot be calculated, while @NA places "NA" in the cell when the value is not available. The function @PI places the value 3.141592653589794 in the cell.

A keyboard *macro* is a predefined sequence of keystrokes (or a user-defined mini-program) that the computer executes when invoked. It is most useful for repetitive tasks or creating sophisticated data input and output sub-routines. The macro usually involves both the entering of data and the invoking of a number of menu commands. (An example of using macros is found in the last example of this chapter.)

Using *command menus* and the keyboard's special *function keys*, you can quickly move around in the spreadsheet and create data and mathematical models and data relationships. Whenever possible let the computer do the work for you. There are two types of data in a spreadsheet: *source data* and *derived data* (or what the spreadsheet's formulas produce). Ideally, a good spreadsheet layout keeps the amount of source data to a minimum while maximizing the use of derived data. Your creative and technical understanding of the spreadsheet software will permit you to use spreadsheets in your agency operations whenever possible.

While the use of spreadsheet packages for standard accounting and budgeting functions in human service agencies are commonly known, other useful applications are also available. In the following pages several examples depict a variety of non-fiscal uses of spreadsheet analysis in human service. First, some applications of spreadsheet programs in direct practice settings are shown. These examples demonstrate graphic display and trend analysis of client functioning measures. Next, an approach to the development and tracking of program performance indicators is provided. A third example shows the use of the spreadsheet capability to model alternatives for program decision-making. The final example demonstrates the creation of an automated service application form in a spreadsheet environment. All of the examples make use of the package, Lotus 1-2-3.

ACCOUNTABILITY AND EVALUATION IN DIRECT PRACTICE

There is an increasing interest in making human service delivery scientifically based. Accountability and evaluation have become increasingly important in direct practice. One significant recent development in direct practice evaluation is the introduction of single subject research methods.

Single subject research provides a set of techniques for experimental manipulation of interventions in a time series with a single client. Typically, this approach involves a combination of baseline and intervention phases and continuous measurement of dependent variables. Single subject research methods have a number of advantages over traditional between-group approaches for use in direct practice. These benefits include simplicity to learn and use, less cost, less intrusiveness, and greater applicability where small caseloads exist or for the study of rare problems. Application of single subject methods to evaluate psychotherapeutic and human service interventions is becoming increasingly widespread (Jayaratne and Levy, 1979; Nelsen, 1981; Bloom and Fischer, 1982; Kazdin, 1982; Berlin, 1983; Bellock and Hersen, 1984; Blythe and Briar, 1985).

While between-group research methods rely heavily on statistical procedures for analysis of data, prevalent methods for analysis of single subject data are primarily visual. Researchers or evaluation-oriented practitioners prepare graphs for visual display of the data which provide the basis for interpretation (Parsonson and Baer, 1978; Bloom and Fischer, 1982).

The increasing emphasis on empirical validation of interventions and the use of single subject research techniques in direct practice has been facilitated by the development of standardized scales for use by workers (Levitt and Reid, 1981). Among the best validated and most widely used scales are those in the Clinical Measurement Package (Hudson, 1982). This package of scales measures depression, self-esteem, marital discord, sexual discord, parent-child relationship problems as seen by parent and child, intrafamilial stress and peer relationship problems. One of the most useful features of these scales is that all are designed with a clinical cutting score, which means that persons scoring 30 or more are believed to be able to benefit from therapeutic intervention. The effectiveness of therapy can be assessed by repetitive administration of these scales, and by plotting scale scores. Computer spreadsheet programs provide a ready vehicle for making such entries, for performing available statistical analyses and for generating plots or graphs to visually display trends in client performance.

Example: Graphic Presentation of Clinical Data

Figure 1 shows scores for a client on two Clinical Measurement Package instruments entered into a spreadsheet layout. In this case, a worker has met with a depressed client for three months and administered the Hudson Generalized Contentment Scale (GCS) and Index of Self Esteem on a weekly basis.

From the spreadsheet entries, the creating of a line graph to display trends in the scale scores becomes a simple procedure. The resulting graph is shown in Figure 2.

```
A1:  'WEEK                                                      READY


         A        B        C        D      E      F      G      H
  1 WEEK      GCS      ISE      CUTTING
  2      1       53       47       30
  3      2       51       49       30
  4      3       44       46       30
  5      4       42       45       30
  6      5       48       45       30
  7      6       43       46       30
  8      7       36       42       30
  9      8       29       40       30
 10      9       24       37       30
 11     10       27       35       30
 12     11       22       34       30
 13     12       17       29       30
 14     13       17       25       30
 15
 16
 17
 18
 19
 20
```

FIGURE 1. Clinical data worksheet

Example: Use of Celeration Line to Determine Change in Trend

A trend or celeration line may be drawn from graphed time-series data to determine if observations in a second phase are a continuation of a trend in the preceding phase (Parsonson and Baer, 1978; Bloom and Fischer, 1982). A celeration line is the best-fitted straight line to show the direction of change in a series of measures. If a celeration line is drawn reflecting a series of measures taken prior to the start of treatment (e.g., baseline phase), then this line may be extended to see whether the measures taken after intervention began continue to follow the same trend as during the baseline period. Therefore, a celeration line helps show whether an upward or downward trend exists in a series of measurements and also allows for the comparison of direction of change in a succeeding treatment phase.

Several approaches have been suggested for drawing a celeration line. The split middle or quartile approach identifies two coordinates on a graph from which to manually draw the line. A more

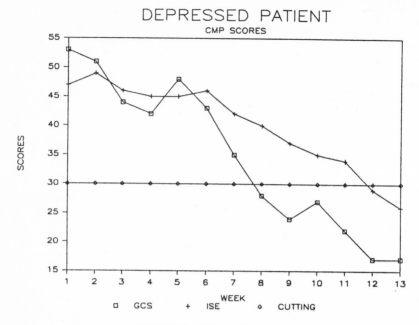

FIGURE 2. Clinical data graph

sophisticated procedure arrives at the placement of the trend line mathematically and involves a method called least squares. A least squares trend line can be calculated from a series of measures and even extended or projected into a later phase of treatment.[1]

The resulting spreadsheet is shown in Figure 3. The expected values column (E) displays a least squares trend line extended to 25 points for whatever values are entered in the baseline (C) column. Data in the baseline column may be changed at will and the new trend line values will be automatically recalculated.

Figure 4 shows how the resulting graph might appear, as produced by the spreadsheet graphics capability.

Example: Testing the Significance of Changes in Trend During Treatment

The statistical significance of changes occurring in the trend line across the treatment phase may be determined, and may be included in a worksheet program. If the hypothesis of no change is true, the

	A	B	C	D	E	F	G	H
1	LEAST SQUARES TREND LINE MATRIX							
2	DATA-PT	DATA-PTSQBASELINE		X-PROD	EXPECTED		TX CUTTING	
3	1	1	58	58	57.64		30	
4	2	4	54	108	57.86		30	
5	3	9	59	177	58.07		30	
6	4	16	65	260	58.29		30	
7	5	25	56	280	58.50		30	
8	6	36	57	342	58.71		30	
9	7	49	59	413	58.93		30	
10	8	64		0	59.14	53	30	
11	9	81		0	59.36	48	30	
12	10	100		0	59.57	42	30	
13	11	121		0	59.79	40	30	
14	12	144		0	60.00	33	30	
15	13	169		0	60.21	57	30	
16	14	196		0	60.43	28	30	
17	15	225		0	60.64			
18	16	256		0	60.86			
19	17	289		0	61.07			
20	18	324		0	61.29			
21	19	361		0	61.50			
22	20	400		0	61.71			
23	21	441		0	61.93			
24	22	484		0	62.14			
25	23	529		0	62.36			
26	24	576		0	62.57			
27	25	625		0	62.79			
28			408	1638				
29								
30		7 N (Number of DATA-PTS)						
31		28 SUM OF DATA-PTS						
32		140 SUM OF DATA-PTS-SQD						
33								
34		196 DENOMINATOR						
35 B=		0.214285 SLOPE						
36 A=		57.42857 INTERCEPT (on Y axis)						

INTERVENTIONS SIGNIFICANTLY DIFFERENT FROM BASELINE (Binomial test)
(1=Significant at .05 level, 0=Not significant)　　　　1

FIGURE 3. Celeration line worksheet

slope of the line constructed for the baseline data should predict the slope of the line during treatment. In other words, since the celeration line represents the midpoint of the baseline scores, half of the treatment scores should also fall above the extrapolated line and half below the line. The probability that a set of scores differs from the expected half-above-and-half-below the trend line may be calculated, using the binomial test (Kazdin, 1982; Bloom and Fischer, 1982). This test of significance may be added to the worksheet and be automatically executed with the entry of time series data. In

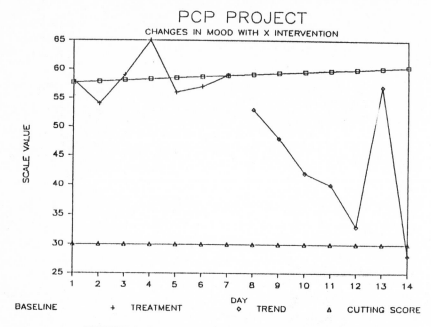

FIGURE 4. Graph of clinical data with celeration line

Figure 3, the results of the binomial test are shown at the bottom of the display. If the number of observation scores below expected values is statistically significant at the .05 level, then a "1" is displayed. If differences are not statistically significant, a "0" is displayed. When new treatment scores are added, the significance of change in trend is automatically redetermined.

PERFORMANCE INDICATORS

Another critical but difficult issue in the human services is how to evaluate the effectiveness of programs. In attempting to conduct program evaluation, an ingredient often missing is a clear criterion of success. One solution to this problem is to provide not an absolute standard, but to use comparisons of similar programs on variables thought to be essential for evaluation. These comparisons might be agency-to-agency, office-to-office, state-to-state, etc., where similar levels of programs are identified. A second approach would be to track performance of a single program over time on a particular indicator. Or, a combination of the two approaches might be utilized. Over a period of time, by watching these comparisons and validating performances with information from program reviews and specific studies, more absolute standards and criteria for effectiveness may be established.

Example: Foster Care Performance Indicators

Figure 5 shows an example of a program indicator that might be used to compare performance in the area of foster care services. This measure is a comparison of the average number of months that foster children have been out of their own homes and in foster care across districts in a state-operated child welfare program. The choice of this indicator is based upon a philosophy of permanency for children and the belief that a comparison of figures showing length of stay in foster care might indicate which districts are implementing permanency planning most effectively.

```
A1: 'GOAL 8: REDUCE TIME IN OUT-OF-HOME CARE                           READY


         A       B    C    D      E       F        G         H
  1 GOAL 8: REDUCE TIME IN OUT-OF-HOME CARE
  2    STANDARD: MEDIAN TIME (MOS) IN SUB-CARE REDUCED 3% FROM PRIOR PERIOD
  3                              Q1-Q2    REDUCTION Q1-Q2      REDUCTION
  4 DIST    Q1 86 Q2 86 Q3 86  % REDUCED  RANK    % REDUCED  RANK
  5 7A       13.6  10.2   6.8    25.00%     1       33.33%      1
  6 2A       14.5  12.7  10.2    12.41%     3       19.69%      2
  7 3        12.3  14.2   12    -15.45%    12       15.49%      3
  8 4         9.2  10.2   8.7   -10.87%     8       14.71%      4
  9 2B       14.4  16.6  14.7   -15.28%    11       11.45%      5
 10 2S        8.4    8    7.6     4.76%     6        5.00%      6
 11 5         6.3   7.2   6.9   -14.29%    10        4.17%      7
 12 1        16.6  18.5    18   -11.45%     9        2.70%      8
 13 2K       10.8   9.6   9.5    11.11%     4        1.04%      9
 14 6        20.1  20.5  20.5    -1.99%     7        0.00%     10
 15 2C        9.5    8    9.2    15.79%     2      -15.00%     11
 16 2T       14.3  16.6  19.1   -16.08%    13      -15.06%     12
 17 7B        8.5    8    10      5.88%     5      -25.00%     13
 18 STATEWIDE 12.2 12.3  11.8    -1.14%              4.43%
 19
 20
```

FIGURE 5. Foster care performance indicator worksheet

The resulting spreadsheet table (shown in Figure 5) highlights the districts making the most progress in reducing the term of stay for children in foster care.

As data for succeeding periods of time become available, these figures may be added to the spreadsheet and new rankings identified. Using the computer spreadsheet capability, a variety of comparisons can easily be made from these data, including raw comparisons of rates between districts, trends for individual districts over time, combined statewide rates and trends, identification of districts falling above and below statewide averages, etc. In addition to the use of tables for presentation of findings, computer graphics may be created to improve the visual impact and meaning of such figures.

BUILDING MODELS TO ASSIST
PROGRAM DECISION-MAKING

Sometimes complex problems are easier to solve if a model can be constructed to test the impact of alternative solutions. Spreadsheet programs allow such models to be created.

Example: Day Care Center Fee Schedule Model

Figure 6 shows an example of the use of spreadsheet software to build a "what if" model. In this example, administrators of a statewide day care licensing function decided that they needed to develop a formula for charging fees for licensing. Previously, this licensing had been done without charge, but because of budget shortfalls, the need existed to recoup sufficient monies from fees to sustain the current staff level.

The model worksheet shown in Figure 6 allows the entry and testing of various combinations of charges for initial licensing fee, initial licensing charge per slot, license renewal fee, and license renewal charge per slot.

Additionally, the model projects costs to varying sizes of day care center, as in the example, for 20, 50, 100, 200, and 300 slots. Varying combinations of charges may be entered into the model. The effect of different formulas on total collections and on the costs to day care centers of various sizes may be seen immediately. From

```
A1:  (C2)                                                           READY


          A        B        C        D        E        F        G        H
 1 DAY CARE CENTER FEE COLLECTION MODEL
 2
 3         200 NEW LICENSES PER YEAR
 4         410 RENEWALS PER YEAR
 5       34000 TOTAL SLOTS IN LICENSED CENTERS
 6                                         PROJECTED COLLECTIONS/YR
 7      $35.00 INITIAL LICENSING FEE                  $7,000.00
 8       $3.00 INITIAL LICENSING CHARGE PER SLOT     $49,756.10
 9      $25.00 LICENSE RENEWAL FEE                   $10,250.00
10       $1.00 LICENSE RENEWAL CHARGE PER SLOT       $34,000.00
11                   TOTAL COLLECTIONS             $101,006.10
12
13
14 COSTS TO CENTERS:
15 NUMBER OF SLOTS         20       50      100      200      300
16 APPLICATIONS        $95.00  $185.00  $335.00  $635.00  $935.00
17 RENEWALS            $45.00   $75.00  $125.00  $225.00  $325.00
18
19
20
```

FIGURE 6. Fee schedule model worksheet

the various worksheet options, the formula can be selected which results in collections of the desired amount yet also appears to be the most equitable and politically feasible.

APPLICATION FORM TEMPLATE

If an agency has eligibility requirements or a sliding fee schedule to apply to applicants for service, spreadsheets provide a capability to automate this process. It is becoming common for large, advanced computer systems in social welfare to provide this capability. With a minimal investment of time and resources, a smaller agency might tailor such a program to its own needs, using spreadsheet software on a microcomputer. Even a large agency might choose to meet the requirements of a specific service through creating such a spreadsheet program. Or further, some of the early development and piloting of a program to eventually be incorporated into a large, main-frame system might be done initially using spreadsheet capabilities.

The scenario for the use of a computerized application form might be this: A client enters the waiting area of an agency and asks for a particular service. A receptionist or intake interviewer loads the spreadsheet application form program into a desk-top micro-computer. As the applicant supplies information, the worker enters the responses into the computer. After each entry, the spreadsheet program may automatically move the cursor to the next input field to prompt the next question from the interviewer and to continue entry. When all the items are answered, the program automatically calculates the applicant's eligibility and fee amounts. Then the program prints a form which includes the information the applicant has supplied, the eligibility and fee status, application "boiler-plate" (i.e., certifications, client rights statements), and lines for needed signatures.

Some of the advantages of this procedure are:

— No costs for design, printing and storage for form stock.
— The only paper handled is the final printed copy of the form.
— Form revisions may be made and implemented without lag time for printing or distribution of forms stock — no wastage of obsolete form stock.
— Data are only entered once, reducing transcription time and copying/keying errors.
— The client sees and approves the exact information acquired by the agency.
— Calculation errors are eliminated.

This sort of spreadsheet program is typically created through the use of "macros." Macros are instructions which pre-identify extended series of keystrokes, saving much operator time and allowing for the creation of relatively complex application programs or templates.

Example: Application Form with Automated Eligibility/Fee Determination

In this example,[2] the form is an application for low-income day care assistance and other social services (i.e., homemaker, day programs for the handicapped). An original menu created just for the program gives the user the option to Add a client, Clear the form, Print the form or Quit (exit) the program. Each of these routines are keyboard macros—sequences of keystrokes which are invoked when the particular menu item is selected. The Add Client routine is an example of an interactive macro. This macro is built to pause in turn at each input field on the form; when the worker completes the entry of a particular item by pressing the ENTER key, the program moves the cell pointer to the next entry field. When entry of information is complete, the program automatically calculates eligibility and fees and re-displays the menu. The worker then may select the print option on the menu to print the completed form ready for the signature.

Figure 7 shows the spreadsheet as it looks after initial loading. The menu is at the top of the page and a portion of the top of first page of the form is also displayed.

Figure 8 shows one of the several tables which the program references for eligibility information for families of different sizes. This is the table for a family with three members. Column B identifies

```
A1:                                                     CMD MENU
ADD  CLEAR  PRINT    QUIT
CLIENT
         A      B      C      D      E       F       G       H    I   J
1                            ELIGIBILITY DECLARATION FOR SOCIAL SERVICES  Form 24
2
3      A 1. Name                     7. Unique I.D. #
4        2.Address                   8. Number in household
5        3.City                      9. I have a Medical Card       Yes
6        4.State & Zip              10. I receive                   AFDC
7        5. Telephone Number        11. I receive                   SSI
8        6.Soc. Sec. #                  Amount
9
10       (If "Yes" is checked in "9", or "10", or "11" above, go to item "E" below
11       AFDC client with a medical card applying for day care)
12
13     B INCOME LISTING: Enter the amount of money received by you, your spouse
14       your household during the most recently completed month.  Omit earnings
15
16       Gross Earnings (including tips)        Railroad Retirement
17       Commissions                            Unemployment Compensation
18       Self-Employment (farm & non-farm)      Workman's Compensation
19       Social Security                        Alimony, Child Support
20       Veteran's Pensions                     Other Income (indicate so
```

FIGURE 7. Initial application form display

```
A1:  U                                                        CMD READY


        A       B        C       D      E      F      G      H   I   J
  161
  162
  163          MAXIMUM    FEE     FEE
  164 FAMILY  COUNTABLE   ONE     TWO
  165 SIZE    INCOME     CHILD  CHILDREN
  166   3         0        0       0
  167            536       9      11
  168            587      14      18
  169            637      19      24
  170            687      26      33
  171            737      33      41
  172            787      41      51
  173            837      49      61
  174            884      58      73
  175            937      67      84
  176            987      77      96
  177           1037      87     109
  178           1087     100     125
  179           1103    9999    9999
  180
```

FIGURE 8. Sample eligibility table

the top figure for a range of countable income. Column C gives the fee when one child is in day care, while column D shows the fee amount for two children.

CONCLUSIONS

One of the newer and more creative ways personal computers are being used in human services is by creating electronic spreadsheets for analyzing data, answering "what if" questions, and modeling decision alternatives. As such, this chapter has defined key concepts agency staff must understand in using any spreadsheet analysis and presented several examples of how spreadsheets could be used in direct practice as well as human service management and administration. As illustrated, computerized spreadsheets can be used to manage and track client and program performance indicators to show trends and areas for concern, as well as make "what-if" projections and model alternatives for program decision-making.

NOTES

1. The least squares trend line program for a spreadsheet and commands for other worksheets shown as examples in this chapter may be obtained from the second author.

2. This program was developed by Jim Shearer of the Utah Department of Social Services. The authors are grateful for his permission to use this example.

REFERENCES

Bellock, A. S. & Hersen, M. (1984). *Research methods in clinical psychology.* New York: Pergamon.

Berlin, S. B. (1983). Single-case evaluation: another version. *Social Work Research and Abstracts, 19*(1), 3-11.

Bloom, M. & Fischer, J. (1982). *Evaluating practice: Guidelines for the accountable professional.* Englewood Cliffs, NJ: Prentice-Hall.

Blythe, B. J. & Briar, S. (1985). Developing empirically based models of practice. *Social Work, 30*, 199-207.

Hudson, W. W. (1982). *The clinical measurement package.* Homewood, IL: Dorsey.

Jayaratne, S. & Levy, R. L. (1979). *Empirical clinical practice.* New York: Columbia University Press.

Kazdin, A. E. (1982). *Single-case research designs: Methods for clinical and applied settings.* New York: Oxford University Press.

Levitt, J. L. & Reid, W. J. (1981). Rapid assessment instruments for practice. *Social Work Research and Abstracts, 17*, 13-20.

Nelson, J. C. (1981). Issues in single-subject research for non-behaviorists. *Social Work Research and Abstracts, 17*(2), 31-37.

Parsonson, B. S. & Baer, D. M. (1978). The analysis and presentation of graphic data. In T. R. Kratochwill (Ed.), *Single subject research: strategies for evaluating change.* New York: Academic Press.

Desktop Publishing for Human Services

Linda D. Iroff

KEYWORDS. Desktop publishing, electronic publishing, page layout

SUMMARY. Computers, especially microcomputers, are helping human service agencies gather and organize an ever-growing amount of information. The new area of desktop publishing can help agencies present that information to clients, funding sources, reporting agencies, and the community, in a clear and easy to understand manner. Desktop publishing can result in professional looking documents at a fraction of the cost of traditional typesetting methods. This paper outlines some of the concepts and benefits of desktop publishing for human services, and points out some of the potential pitfalls.

INTRODUCTION

Like most organizations, human service agencies are plagued with an overabundance of paper. Information comes in fast and in too great a quantity to be handled effectively, especially if the information must be processed and reformulated before moving to its next destination. There are internal memos and reports, external correspondence, forms and informational brochures for clients, formal reports and grant proposals for funding sources, and so forth. The effectiveness of all this information is often directly related to its readability (Rapp & Poertner, 1986).

Until recently, there have been two ways in which an organization can produce this paper: internally, by typewriters or computers,

Linda D. Iroff is a computer support specialist for the College of Arts and Sciences, Cornell University, Ithaca, NY 14853 and a freelance writer for computer magazines.

69

or externally, by graphic designers and typesetters. Internally produced material has the benefit of being quick and inexpensive to produce, although limitations of output choices can reduce the effectiveness of the material. Some documents must include photographs, charts, and artwork requiring complex layout and design pasteup. Professional services for such work can be expensive, and require a significant amount of lead time.

There is now a third alternative. The new field of desktop publishing allows human service organizations to create professional looking documents quickly and inexpensively with a microcomputer and laser printer (Gray, 1986; Needle, 1987; Mariani, 1987). Desktop publishing can be especially useful for producing clear and understandable forms for clients, and for professional looking reports and proposals.

WHAT IS DESKTOP PUBLISHING AND HOW DOES IT WORK?

Desktop publishing[1] is an editorial design technology based on the use of a microcomputer, appropriate software, and a high resolution printer (such as a laser printer) to produce camera ready copy, i.e., copy that is directly ready for reproduction by a printing press.

In the traditional publishing process, the author or editor gathers the text and images (graphs, tables, photographs, illustrations) for a single package that might be a report, a flyer, a brochure, or a book. Text and graphics are then turned over to someone who provides the design and technical directions for turning the document into a printed product.

In desktop publishing, the microcomputer is used to not only produce the text, but also to complete the full design of the publication. It allows for the interactive combination of text and graphics, and gives the user extensive control as to how they will be placed on each page, along with headlines and other page decorations. Usually, some element of WYSIWYG ("What You See Is What You

---

[1]The term was coined in 1984 by Paul Brainerd of Aldus Corporation, maker of one of the first page layout programs for the Macintosh.

Get'') is involved, i.e., the screen gives a fairly accurate representation of how the document will appear when printed.

The process of creating camera ready copy usually involves several steps and several programs depending on the complexity of the final product. Text is first produced with a word processing program. Some formatting may take place at this time—fonts, styles (bold, italic, etc.), tabs, indents—while other formatting is done with the page layout program (see below). A good operating principle is to keep the word processing simple and avoid the attempt to "design" at this stage.

A wide variety of graphics programs can be used. Charting programs can accept raw data or take the output from a data base or spreadsheet and produce line, bar, or pie charts. A painting program can be used to produce freeform artwork, while a drawing or drafting program is usually more suitable for more structured artwork and line art, such as diagrams. Existing graphics such as maps or photographs can also be read into the computer using an optical scanner. Commercially produced "clip art" (pictures in electronic form) exists for those with no artistic skill.

The text and graphic elements are combined with a page layout or desktop publishing program. Text can be placed in multiple columns and can automatically flow to succeeding pages as needed. A user can create new text or edit existing text, add style or format changes, and create headers and footers that contain the same information on each page (or alternate for left and right hand pages). Text can be justified on the left, right or both sides, line and character spacing ("leading and kerning") can be varied, and words automatically hyphenated. Headlines can be added to different stories, rules placed between columns, and other graphic elements added.

Graphics can be placed anywhere on the page, with text flowing around it. Pictures can be scaled or cropped to fit the available space. Lines and boxes with different shapes and thicknesses can be drawn to separate sections or surround graphics. Shapes can be filled with patterns or shaded with varying levels of grey for attractive backgrounds.

Many programs allow you to set up grids that make it easier to line up different elements. Some allow you to create style sheets so you can use a consistent style for several documents, and may even include some sample layouts to help a novice get started.

Usually, all this layout is done visually, with some semblance of WYSIWYG. However, sometimes the exact layout of a page can only be seen in a reduced size that may not allow editing or rearrangement. The low resolution of the CRT relative to the printer also necessitates test printing in order to make fine adjustments. Printing is usually done on a laser printer, although higher quality print is available from some service bureaus (see below).

SETTING UP A DESKTOP PUBLISHING SYSTEM

The startup costs for desktop publishing are generally quoted at about $10,000 (Hart, 1987), but this amount can be misleading. A desktop publishing system need not be a dedicated system; the computer and printer may be used for many other tasks, such as general word processing, accounting, budgeting, data base record keeping, etc. Many human service agencies, in fact, now have microcomputer systems for these and other tasks (Doucette, 1985), and the costs of adding desktop publishing can be relatively low. The following gives some idea of what hardware and software are appropriate.

The Apple Macintosh was the system on which desktop publishing was first introduced. A minimal system would include a Macintosh SE with 1 MByte RAM and a 20 MByte hard disk. On the IBM compatible side, an AT compatible or System/2 computer is preferred, since the earlier PC and XT models may be too slow. A graphics adapter, mouse, hard disk, and minimum of 1 MB RAM are also required. Enhanced graphics adapters for the IBM are preferable. More memory and large screen monitors that can show at least one full 8 1/2 by 11 inch page are useful additions for both IBM and Mac (Felici, 1987).

The Apple LaserWriter was the first printer to use PostScript, a programming language for describing page output, that made desktop publishing possible (Strehlo & Felici, 1987). It is capable of producing full page graphics at 300 dpi (dots per inch). Non-PostScript printers laser printers can produce text at 300 dpi, but graphics may be restricted to half or quarter page at 300 dpi (or full page at 150 dpi), unless more memory is added to the printer. Special effects such as rotated text and graduated grey scales may also be unavailable. Limited memory can also restrict the number of typefaces used in one document. Laser printers include a number of built-in fonts; more fonts can be added through software or plug-in cartridges.

The 300 dots per inch of a laser printer may be adequate for most uses, but a formal report, a book, journal or magazine may require a more professional look. Many professional phototypesetting machines (such as Linotronic and Compugraphic) can now accept output from microcomputer page layout programs and produce output at up to 2600 dpi. If this higher quality is required, the laser printer can act as a proofing machine, letting a user know exactly how output will look before sending it to the typesetter. Phototypesetting equipment is expensive (tens of thousands of dollars), but typesetting services will produce output from disks for $6 to $12 per page (Kobler, 1988).

In choosing software, the key issue is compatibility between the programs that you use to create the text and graphics, and the page layout program you use to put them together. On the Macintosh, this is often not as much of a problem, since there are defined standards for how text and graphics are stored on the computer. It is generally easy to get information into the page layout program, although text formatting is not always maintained, and some new graphics standards for scanned images may not be supported by older page layout programs.

The issue is somewhat more complex for IBM compatibles. Many desktop publishing programs for the IBM run under a specific operating environment,[2] such as *Microsoft Windows*, *GEM* or *OS/2 Presentation Manager*. Any other programs that run under the same environment should be able to exchange information as appropriate. In addition, most page layout programs have a list of popular word processing and graphics programs from which they can accept data.

---

[2]An *operating environment* provides a standard interface (usually Macintosh-like) for any program that operates under that environment. Similar tasks in different programs are done the same way, making it easier to learn new programs. Data transfer between programs is also facilitated.

The type of documents to be produced also play an important role in choosing an appropriate page layout program. Some programs (e.g., PageMaker for both Macintosh and PC) are better suited for laying out individual pages which vary greatly, such as an informational brochure for clients, a short newsletter, posters, etc.; others (Ventura Publisher and Quark XPress) perform best on longer, more consistent documents, such as an annual report or grant proposal. But as in any type of software, no one program can have every feature; the user must decide which has the best mix of features for his/her needs.

A user must also be sure the page layout program is compatible with the laser printer. Fortunately, many programs, printers, and even typesetting machines are standardizing on PostScript. However, the situation may become more clouded with the appearance of ''PostScript clones'' which may reduce compatibility (Sorensen, 1987), and of QuickDraw laser printers (Felici, 1988). It is also worth noting that many new word processing programs are incorporating desktop publishing features (Pepper, 1988; Farber, 1987).

CAVEATS

Desktop publishing programs are not omnipotent; they usually lack such standard word processing features as outlining, paragraph sorting and footnoting. Users can set up a form letter in a page layout program, but mailmerge features are not available to integrate the letter with a list of names. And while the layout programs can be used to help design a form, laser printers will not print on multi-part carbon copy forms, which must still be filled out by hand or typewriter.

A more important concern is one of training. Desktop publishing may require a four-fold learning process. After first learning the word processing and graphics programs for creating the initial text and pictures, the user must then learn the mechanics of running the layout program, which in itself may be a time-consuming task given the feature-laden complexity of these programs. Third, the would-be desktop publisher must become familiar with much of the terminology and concepts involved in publishing in order to use these programs effectively. And finally, the user should gain a basic knowledge of good design principles (see below).

Fortunately, local universities and computer stores often sponsor desktop publishing seminars and workshops, and in larger cities, professional training centers hold classes. Expect to pay from $100 to $300 for a day of training (Perdue, 1988). For those who prefer self-learning, there are a plethora of books, video and audio cassettes, and disk-based training packages available, though they may be of mixed utility (Eckhardt, 1988).

No matter how the training is accomplished, it may take some time to get up to speed on a page layout system. Even an experienced computer user will need time to learn the publishing concepts involved. The first few documents will probably take longer to produce than by traditional means, but time savings will quickly be realized as the user becomes familiar with the process, and as desktop-published document designs are reused (as in a monthly newsletter, or a form or brochure that needs modification).

DESIGN ISSUES

A page layout program does not make a user into a good designer. In fact, it becomes much easier to create a badly designed document, which can detract from the message one is trying to convey (Greitzer, 1986; Burns & Venit, 1987).

A basic tenet, especially for beginners, is to keep it simple. Stick to one typeface family, using different sizes, italics, boldface, etc., for needed emphasis, and use a minimum of graphic elements. Too many fonts and graphics can be distracting to the reader.

On the other hand, a document's design can be too boring. The use of subheadings to break up large blocks of text, and white space can clearly delineate where one article ends and the next starts. Visual emphasis can also be added to important elements.

Be aware, however, that it is very easy to end up spending a great deal of time adjusting the layout of a page, and thus have proportionally less time to make sure the editorial content is worthwhile and accurate.

More information on laying out attractive documents can be obtained from a book on basic design. There are also a number of magazines that cover the burgeoning desktop publishing industry. In a positive move, many publishing programs now include manuals on the principles of design.

CONCLUSION

Human service providers can garner many advantages from entering the field of desktop publishing. First and foremost is the ability to lower the out-of-pocket costs of producing necessary printed materials. At a modest estimate, a single page of professionally produced publication can cost $45 just for design, layout, and typography. At this rate, only 200 pages of output will pay for the basic technology.

More importantly, the gates are open for putting the best word-and-image power to work on all the message output of the agency. Making forms easy to use can have a strong positive impact on workers and clients, as well as managers and supervisors. Financial and program reports for monthly board meetings can become more readable, and daily agency life can become more "user friendly" through the generation of miniposters and graphics that communicate new messages and continuing themes.

Time is a valuable commodity in any organization. The great advantage of desktop publishing over other methods is the potential for cutting the time from when a text is written to when it is distributed as a printed product. It becomes easier to try out several different designs for a publication without losing weeks in the process, thus better choices can be made and major mistakes avoided. All too often the decision is made that something is "good enough" when there simply is no more time or money available to make things right.

Finally, desktop publishing opens up a powerful resource for development of inexpensive but professional looking materials aimed at the fundraising needs of organizations. The polished look can reflect positively on the organization, resulting in more effective fundraising.

REFERENCES

Burns, D. & Venit, S. (1987, October 13). What's Wrong with this Page? *PC Magazine*, pp. 173-175.

Doucette, J. (1985). Directory of Microcomputer Software in the Human Services. Portland, ME: Computer Consulting and Programming Associates. p. 175.

Eckhardt, R. C. (1988, March). The Self-Taught Publisher. *Publish*, pp. 60-63.

Farber, D. (1987, September 14). FullWrite: Word Processor Breaks the Mold. *Macintosh Today*, p. 44.

Felici, J. (1987, May), Screen Tests. *Publish*, pp. 50-57.

Felici, J. (1988, February). Personal Laser Printer. *Publish*, pp. 68-70.

Greitzer, J. (1986, November/December). Design Police. *Publish*, pp. 48-53.

Gray, P. J. (1986). Desktop Publishing. *Evaluation Practice, 10* (3), 40-49.

Hart, R. (1987, July). The Big Bundle: PC Turnkey Systems. *Publish*, pp. 52-59.

Kobler, J. (1988, July). Check Please. *Publish*, pp. 58-61.

Pepper, J. (1988, June 21). Word Perfect 5.0 Seamlessly Melds Text, Graphics. *PC Week*, pp. 93-98.

Perdue, L. (1988, March). Hired Education. *Publish*, pp. 55-59.

Mariani, J. (1987, October 26). Desktop Publishing Systems Save Typesetting Work, Costs for Agencies. *Syracuse Post Standard*, p. D1.

Needle, D. (1987, January/February). Resourceful by Nature. *Publish*, pp. 82-85.

Rapp, C. A. & Poertner, J. (1986). The Design of Data-based Management Reports. *Admin. in Social Work, 10* (4), 53-64.

Sorensen, K. (1987, October 12). PostScript Clones Point to Faster Printers. *Macintosh Today*, p. 25.

Strehlo, K. & Felici, J. (1987, November). The Great PostScript Printer Race. *Publish*, pp. 50-61.

Selecting a Computer-Based System to Assist Fund-Raising and Development Operations

Sandra R. Simon
William H. Button

KEYWORDS. Fund-raising, donor database, personalization, fund accounting, community organization, computerized development system

SUMMARY. Increasingly, non-profit organizations and agencies must turn to the private sector to raise money to finance their work, and to increase the scope of their services. Computer software is available to assist and enhance organizational development efforts involving direct mail, "events," and broadcast appeals. Social Work professionals may be responsible for selecting software systems for their agencies. What functions should such software perform? What criteria should it meet? The software should contain features that support each stage of a development cycle, manage

---

Sandra R. Simon, MSW, PhD, has a Master's Degree in Social Welfare and a Doctoral Degree in Developmental Biochemistry. As this volume goes to press, she is starting a position with the Texas Department of Human Resources in Austin. She previously worked as a computer consultant to non-profit organizations on Long Island. Her interest is in educational process to expand access to and understanding of technological advance.

William H. Button, PhD, has a Doctoral Degree in Sociology. He is an Associate Professor in the School of Social Welfare, State University of New York at Stony Brook. In addition, he has worked for many years as a computer consultant to non-profit organizations in the New York metropolitan area. His interest is in organizational structure, and in the integration of computer technology into social service agencies.

The expert editorial assistance of Kristina Hansen, MSW, is gratefully acknowledged.

mailing lists, provide financial and fund-accounting functions, produce letters and other communications, and generate statistics and reports for management control. Each of these functions is examined in some detail, as considerations to bear in mind when evaluating systems are discussed.

INTRODUCTION

Social Service agencies increasingly depend upon community financial support for their programmatic and capital needs. During recent lean years, planning, implementation, and management of Fund Raising and Financial Development activities have become critical functions facing agency personnel.

We contend that Social Workers with strong Community Organization skills can play a critical role in the agency's Fund Raising and Development activities. Communicating the organization's mission, needs and accomplishments can generate financial support among individuals, and community and corporate groups. Advocacy for the services urgently needed by the agency's targeted population can take place in many forums. A base of moral commitment can be built among identified coalitions and interest groups prepared to respond to challenges and opportunities that arise. Individuals outraged by injustice, indifference and neglect may respond to requests for financial support and volunteer time on behalf of those truly disenfranchised. The knowledgeable Community Organizer will understand how to mobilize community support by skillfully documenting needs for expansion and intensification of services. Where public policy falls short of meeting human needs, the Social Worker Organizer will know how, when and whom to involve in carefully devised strategies for seeking change and generating financial support from the community.

This chapter will focus on the Fund Raising process as an emerging component of Community Organization, and emphasize the numerous ways in which micro-computer software can enhance the productivity of Fund Raising efforts. Affordable computer hardware and software systems now abound. It is no longer necessary to pencil donor giving histories on 3″ × 5″ cards, alphabetically filed in trays. Impersonal, encoded 4-up labels produced by a local Service Bureau and applied to "Dear Friend" letters can no longer be counted on to elicit a generous response. Xeroxed or mimeographed, hand-addressed receipts need no longer be the typical acknowledgement that modest donors receive. Volunteers need no longer be involved in endless unskilled clerical tasks; they can be redirected toward sophisticated solicitation efforts.

As in other areas of agency administration and operation, we believe the time has come to use micro-computers to enhance this activity.

THE FUND-RAISING CYCLE

Fund Raising Management, a publication serving the fund raising and financial development industry, frequently includes articles about computer-based fund-raising systems. An issue (Sept. 1985) briefly described the products of 53 vendors serving every conceivable segment of the fund raising market. Prices ranged from $375,000 for on-line mainframe systems to as little as $495 for a system operating on a dual-disk drive personal computer. Twenty-two of the software systems were priced between $5,000 and $15,000.

How can a social agency faced with a critical task—fund-raising—and a new technology—microcomputer hardware and software—determine what products are best? How can one decide among the products offered? One can begin by thinking about what functions the software should perform. It might seem that a good word-processing program with mail-merge capability could satisfy one's direct-mail appeal needs. However, an analysis of the tasks involved reveals that more extensive software support is needed at virtually every stage of the fund-raising process.

Development efforts, regardless of the scope of their goals or their duration, all move through the same sequence of stages. These are (1) campaign planning and project design; (2) initiation of the project; (3) donor response; (4) donor acknowledgement and receipting; (5) donation and fund accounting; and (6) feedback and analysis. Ideally, development software should perform functions that serve at each stage of the process. Let us briefly examine some of the tasks involved in each of these stages.

1. Campaign Planning and Project Design

Fund-raising efforts begin with forward planning, often extending over several years, consisting of a variety of campaigns, or major efforts. Each campaign needs to reflect a thorough understanding of the demographics and giving histories of specific segments of the donor population. What previous appeals brought these donors into the fold? How do they identify with the agency's mission? What financial support can be expected from them? To increase the donor base, what prospective groups should be addressed? How?

Within each campaign there will be one or more specific projects. At the point of project design further questions must be answered. What are the project's financial goals? Costs? What is the time frame? What features will characterize this appeal? What materials and literature must be prepared? Should outreach efforts be directed toward new, potential donors?

Successful campaigns and projects are designed with careful attention to detail. The effectiveness of written appeals hinges on the ability to segment donor and prospect pools wisely, and to direct to each targeted segment appropriately motivating, timely, personalized communications.

2. Initiation of the Project

The project is initiated when the first publicity and/or direct mail appeals are released. At this point, donor acknowledgement devices should be prepared, and be ready for use. Procedures should have been established to handle donor responses and to begin accumulating financial and demographic information for statistical evaluation. If this is a particularly large and costly mailing, alternative formats may be tested prior to full scale commitment to one format.

3. Donor Response

As responses are received, they must be categorized; donations must be dated, recorded, and properly accounted for. Fund Raisers must be able to analyze demographic and financial details of the response in order to determine how the appeal is being received. If necessary, "second wave" written or personal communications must be initiated.

As donor acknowledgement and receipting continue, donor records must be updated, to provide information for future projects and campaigns. How many new donors were there; how many donors moved into Membership status as a reflection of increased levels of giving; which large donors failed to respond?

4. Donor Acknowledgement and Receipting

Donors must receive timely, appropriate acknowledgement of their donations, and receipts. Special letters must be sent to recognize first-time donors, to those who gave large contributions, to donors of funds for specific purposes, and to other special groups. Donors who do not wish to receive acknowledgement or receipts must be so categorized, and respected. Any premiums or merchandise associated with the appeal must be shipped.

5. Donations and Fund Accounting

Money received must be posted correctly, so that proper accounting records are maintained. Gifts earmarked by donors for special purposes must be credited to designated funds, with appropriate receipts. Audit trails must be created, assuring that for all funds received there is accurate accounting.

6. Feedback and Analysis

As soon as responses begin to accumulate, information about the project's performance must be gathered for management review.

Project responses must be examined and analyzed in light of financial, demographic and response rate information. What proportion of the target segments responded? On what date after the mail drop did revenues surpass the project cost? What was the largest gift, the number of gifts, the average gift? How does this response compare with other projects in prior years? How many donors increased their support? How fruitful were various prospect lists? How many new donors, new members, new pledgers resulted from the project? What range of donations came from each group? Were media expenses justified? Did donors in larger gift categories respond as anticipated? If merchandise or premiums were offered, was this profitable?

Detailed analysis of every campaign and related project is essential in planning future fund-raising activities and development operations.

SELECTING A COMPUTER SYSTEM

Developmental personnel should evaluate software in terms of its facilities for supporting all phases of the fund-raising cycle. We suggest you examine how well the software fulfills the criteria outlined in the following seven areas:

1. Mailing List Management and Control
2. Control and Integration of Financial Operations
3. Organization and Management of Daily Operations
4. Project and Campaign Management and Control
5. Flexibility and Features of Out-going Document Production
6. Documentation, Training, Support, Program Updates and Service
7. Accommodation for Growth

We will examine each of these areas in some detail. (See Table I for a brief synopsis of considerations.)

1. Mailing List Management and Control

Effective management of an organization's mailing lists—the data bases of donors and prospects—is one of the most important requirements that a computerized fund-raising system must satisfy. When evaluating systems, look at (1) the number and nature of

Considerations In Selecting A Fund-Raising System

1. Mailing List Management and Control
   - Number and nature of fields available
   - Can fields be defined with your vernacular?
   - How are duplicate names found?
   - How are account codes created?
   - Detailed reports about donors/prospects, and changes in their activity
   - Facilities for controlled purging of non-donors

2. Control and Integration of Financial Operations
   - Can system create designated sub-funds as needed?
   - Can system integrate with General Ledger?
   - Forced reconciliation of funds with deposits before posting
   - Extensive daily, weekly, and periodic reports of donor activity
   - Keeps appropriately extensive donor giving history
   - Automatic integration of gift information into donor data bases
   - Facilities for handling: - pledges
                              - merchandise for sale or incentive
   - Rigorous audit trails

3. Organization and Management of Daily Operations
   - Daily key-in time to handle donations and prepare receipts
   - Key-in time required to maintain/update data bases and files
   - Details of: - mail processing routines
                - letter-preparation and storage facilities
                - merchandise management process
   - Ease of obtaining donor records as hard copy or on-line

4. Project and Campaign Management and Control
   - Extent of data (numbers of fields; field size; field customization) that can be stored in each account record
   - Extent of segmentation available for targeting defined groups
   - Ease of obtaining information about changes in donor/prospect involvement
   - Detailed, timely reports about: - campaigns
                                    - specific fund-raising projects and sub-funds
                                    - merchandise for sale or premiums
                                    - pledge programs
                                    - involvement of major donors

5. Flexibility and Features of Out-going Document Production
   - Extent of personalization of any communications with data base information
   - Facilities for: - various output forms
                    - various printers
   - Details of performance during long print runs

6. Documentation, Training, Support, Program Updates and Service
   - Extent of training available
   - Well-written, well-indexed documentation and manuals
   - Availability of: - hot-line support
                     - program updates

7. Accommodation for Growth.
   - Maximum number of names data bases can handle
   - Other ceilings: numbers of financial transactions, number of years of donor history retained, etc.
   - Facilities for re-installation in larger hardware.

TABLE I

discrete items of information (fields) which can be stored regarding each donor account, and (2) the flexibility of the system in adapting to the vernacular and categorization schemes for distinguishing among donor groups. Powerful programs store upwards of 150 discrete items of information for each donor account code.

The extent to which the system permits personalization and segmentation is largely a matter of the size and scope of the information maintained in the donor account data base. A satisfactory system should store enough information to assist you in *improving* your communication with donors; it should never create an impersonal barrier between you and your community.

How does the system detect duplicate names? How effectively this is done will, in part, relate to the method used to uniquely identify individual donor accounts. Some systems use arbitrary, serialized numbers; others generate *matchcodes* from components of the donor's name, ZIP and street address, etc. Effective matchcodes make it possible to scan the database, alphabetically or geographically, to extract identical or very similar account codes for individual review. Such a system will facilitate finding duplicates, or different members of the same household entered into the list. One should then have the option of consolidating these individual accounts and merging both demographic and accounting information.

The system should easily provide "hard copy" reports and/or on-screen information describing a wide variety of changes in the data base of donor/prospect accounts. For example, Fund Raising Management need to know, on at least a monthly basis, numbers of new names, new donors, new pledgers, new members, and where merchandise is offered, new customers. The system should facilitate segmenting on these new relationships to extend organizational involvement.

The system must track and indicate individuals who are continually unresponsive to appeals, and provide easy facilities for purging them from the list, when a decision is made to do so. It should also "protect" other non-donors with whom you want to communicate—public officials, community leaders, etc.—from being purged from the list.

The system should also automatically accommodate donors who do not wish to receive mailings, receipts, and the like.

2. Control and Integration
of Financial Operations

The organization's Controller or Chief Financial Officer, along with the Development Director, should examine how the fund-raising system is "integrated" with standard accounting functions. From the perspective of internal control of funds, contributions are vital revenues that must be accounted for in ways which meet auditable standards. The system should be integrated with the organization's General Ledger system, providing reports of revenues received on a daily, weekly, monthly and annual basis. The system should "force" reconciliation of funds received with bank deposits, prior to posting to donor accounts.

A powerful system should be flexible enough to permit creating as many designated funds as may be needed, to manage donations to specific funds in a manner similar to that used for general donations.

How does the system manage donor accounts, and capture information that is necessary to relate funds received to specific donors? While most accounting systems provide This Year-Prior Year comparisons for "accounts receivable," fund raisers clearly need more information covering a longer time frame. The system should retain relevant data, such as the dates, amounts, and frequency of donations for prior years, and the date and amount of the largest gift ever made. In addition to "giving history," this information may have implications for future development efforts. The need for easy access to this sort of information, in fact, may be one of the main reasons to purchase a computer system!

Integration Between Donations
and Mailing List Data Base

Computerized fund raising programs vary in the manner in which they integrate donations received into the permanent data base of donor records. How much of this process is "automatic" and how much of it must be done manually on a donor-by-donor basis after gifts are recorded? This will have an enormous impact upon the amount of time necessary to keep the data base current.

What options are available with respect to receipting and letters of appreciation and recognition? How are these communications personalized? Can they be designed to differentiate between gifts for general support and those for designated funds? Does the system indicate first-time donors and donors of large gifts? These, and other, indications of significant commitment, should receive special responses (Meyer, 1985).

An effective system should guarantee that each step in the acknowledgement process has actually been taken for every donation received.

For organizations utilizing pledges as a source of continuing support, the system must monitor and respond to those fulfilling or defaulting on such pledges. Find out how these various functions are performed and managed, as well as how flexible and "automatic" the operations really are.

Strategic considerations of fund-raising include building coalitions among diverse groups whose involvement with the organization may vary in significant ways. Specific campaigns or projects may be aimed at different groups. The computer system must provide information about prospects' and donors' responses to these various undertakings. Only with this pool of information can fundraising personnel evaluate the motivational effectiveness of each project, and their overall development strategy. Prepare a "wish list" of information and relationships that you need for analytical purposes, and present it to vendors whose products you are considering.

3. Organization and Management of Daily Operations

A computerized system will have considerable impact on day-to-day operations of the development program. It will significantly change the work of fund raising personnel as it enhances the contribution this department makes to the organization. When evaluating systems one should critically examine what the system will require in terms of staff time and resources, supplies, mailing procedures, additional office equipment, etc.

How much "keying-in" time is required on a daily basis to take advantage of the system's capabilities? Building and maintaining a donor/member/prospect data base of high quality will be an ongoing task. The ease of performing file maintenance operations will affect the amount of staff time that will be needed. How much time is needed for routine daily response entry and receipting? The effective system should increase the productivity of the development office, but will rarely reduce staffing needs.

How does the system provide means for quality assurance in processing mail? A well-designed system will require structured off-line and on-line procedures for handling batches of mail received. An efficient system will involve different batching routines, so that mail received in response devices with donor account numbers can be handled in different ways than batches of "white mail." Similarly, pledge payments, merchandise orders, contributions to special funds, or letters requesting information, etc., should be handled through specific routing procedures.

Maintaining a library of letters and response devices will be an ongoing activity. A computerized system will certainly contain word processing capabilities, and should provide flexible means for inserting pertinent donor data base material, on a donor-by-donor basis, into all communications, for purposes of personalization.

As new information is learned about donors, the system should have facilities for generating appropriate change/update screens to introduce this data.

It should be possible to retrieve, display and print out an entire donor record easily, as needed. This will facilitate staff responses to donor inquiries. It should also be possible to reprint individual receipts for donors who may have misplaced or destroyed their original copies.

For the organization that distributes premiums or offers merchandise for sale, the system must perform a variety of additional functions. It should manage all phases of the merchandise or premium fulfillment process. It should maintain an accurate inventory of a wide variety of items, produce picking sheets and shipping labels, handle back-order situations, and account for all money transactions associated with merchandise. It should have facilities for sending debit and credit letters, as needed. It should be capable of maintaining appropriate sales tax accounts. The status of customer orders should also be available, on-line. Where merchandise sales are undertaken to generate revenues, the system should provide a variety of reports which indicate the relative volume and profitability of the different items offered.

4. Project and Campaign Management and Control

To assess a system's potential for enhancing management and control of projects and campaigns, one should examine (1) the extent of information about donors and prospects that can be retained in the data base, (2) facilities for segmentation, (3) responsiveness to donor changes, and (4) statistical and analytical reports generated about individual fund-raising operations.

Information. Some criteria to consider in evaluation of information captured and stored in the data bases have been described in the section on mailing list management. One should also examine the number and kinds of data categories that are available for customization, both to describe and to segment the various lists. Many organizations make extensive use of special events. It may be important to classify a donor with respect to such activities. (Loykovich, 1985) Also, an organization may need to designate donors in terms of the source which brought them onto the list (Katz, 1985).

If intensive donor profile studies are to be conducted, the amount of demographic data which the list can capture beyond the usual giving history and zip code areas will be important (Sanders, 1985). Organizations incurring media expenses in connection with fund raising efforts may need to relate response to broadcast industry market areas. It may also be important to indicate staff or volunteers responsible for specific efforts. The system should be able to capture these types of information, and to segment the list with respect to these fields.

Segmentation. The system should provide flexible, fast, powerful facilities for segmenting groups of donors and/or prospects, based upon specifically-defined criteria. Programs vary widely with respect to their segmentation procedures and capabilities; needs of different agencies also vary. Evaluate systems in terms of your own organization's needs.

"Segmentation" of the data list means that the system can "pull out" groups based upon specified criteria. The first level of segmentation concerns those groups within the data base that must be separated into mutually exclusive categories, for fund-raising purposes. A special donor who gave a wheelchair van worth $50,000 three years ago, for example, should never receive a routine letter for this year's "dollar-a-month" appeal.

Beyond this level, how extensive should further select requests be? A system limited to five or six levels of segmentation will be able to pinpoint specific groups far less effectively than one with a larger number of select specifications. Generally, the overall size of your lists will determine how critical this is: larger lists require more select options than smaller lists. In addition, efforts which extend beyond one locality or Standard Metropolitan Statistical area may require more select layers. Such fund-raising operations may need systems that support ten or more levels of selection in order to pinpoint specific groups effectively.

Responsiveness to Donor Changes. Computer-based fund raising is a dynamic process. The power of a particular system is in large measure related to how effectively it keeps operators and managers aware of changes. How readily one can respond to these changes will be a function of (1) how the system handles incoming mail and (2) the speed with which important changes in donor status are brought to the attention of system operators. A system should alert operators as donations are processed if, as a result of a gift or communication, something important has changed. For example, as a consequence of an increased level of giving, a donor may have moved "automatically" into a membership category. The system should alert the operator at the point of data entry to that change, so that a special membership response document will be sent.

Reports. The range of available reports — along with their structure, flexibility, and comprehensiveness — will determine the value of the system in providing you with management information. Reports should generate daily, detailed information about the effectiveness of designated projects and campaigns. For an important direct mail appeal, for example, one should be able to see, every day, the volume and nature of the response. This data will facilitate making decisions about follow-up appeals, personal phone calls, increased media expenditures, etc. The system should also produce reports comparing current response with previous campaign pro-files. A wide variety of different reports will help one to analyze fund-raising efforts, and to evaluate any outside consultant or list broker services.

In addition to campaign and project statistics, fund raising direc-tors need reports describing the donor/prospect list, on a monthly basis. Name acquisition and attrition should be clearly delineated, with respect to donor giving levels. Pledge performance should be monitored on a continuing basis. Similarly, sales reports should provide information about the profitability of every item offered for sale.

Of critical concern are reports describing the performance of large donors. Contributions from this group to specific projects, as well as the frequency, amount, and average donation of this group must be readily available for careful review.

Finally, the system should provide comprehensive report facili-ties for managing each special project and campaign effort as inten-sively as the general fund-raising operation.

5. Flexibility and Features of Out-Going Document Production

The increasing volume of direct mail reaching the average Amer-ican household makes it ever more difficult for fund raisers to create messages that will recruit new support. One must (1) maximize appropriate personalization, and (2) avoid, whenever possible, that telltale sign of a mass mailing—the Cheshire label, incorrectly ad-dressed. A computer-based fund raising system must offer great flexibility in preparing creative, attractive communications that speak directly to the prospect or donor.

The system should support personalization through the integra-tion of data base information into any communications prepared with the word-processing component. It should be possible, for ex-ample, to thank a donor for a gift of a specific amount, in response to a specific appeal, applied, as requested, to specific funds.

The system should support the preparation of a wide variety of output documents, through the use of a range of design formats. All systems will generate a personalized letter on standard 8 1/2" × 11" letterhead. A powerful system should also be capable of generating personalized receipts for donors, "bounceback" donation forms, and the like, during the same print pass in which a "thank you" letter is prepared. The system should also be able to use the wide range of composite forms available, that tear apart into various component mailing and response devices.

The system should also support personalizing and printing special forms, such as membership cards, Rolodex cards, and, of course, labels. Where merchandise is being sold, the system should generate shipping labels, merchandise picking lists, and credit and debit notices.

The system must also produce personalized correspondence of a quality that is satisfactory for important larger donors. Both the word-processing facilities and the printers should be evaluated in terms of this need.

Printing outgoing documents is time-consuming. Multi-user and multi-tasking systems, which permit long print runs to proceed while other activities continue at the computer, may significantly increase the productivity of fund-raising operations.

How does the system handle interruptions of long print runs? It should not be necessary to restart the print routine. This involves needless expense, duplication, and time. An effective system should be able to restart a print routine at the point where it was interrupted.

Printers critically affect output appearance and flexibility. Investigate the range and variety of output which the program-printer interface will support. Laser printers offer great speed and design options. Fast, high quality dot matrix printers also support a wide range of options, at reasonable cost. Some organizations may need more than one printer. A system should support the addition of more and/or different types of printers as needed.

6. Documentation, Training, Support, Program Updates and Service

When selecting a system, one must also ask questions about documentation, training, support, program updates, and service. Some vendors of fund-raising programs sell both their software and the hardware on which it will run. These vendors may service the hardware, or may refer you to other maintenance companies.

Organizations who have been using service bureaus or other computer systems should inquire about services to "convert" their data for automatic input into the new system.

In evaluating relative costs for software, it is important to inquire about training. Training may be offered at the vendor's headquarters or "on-site" at your location, using your equipment. Understanding a system and using it to full potential will take a considerable period of time. However, initial training should familiarize development staff and operators with all features of the program in all phases of operation.

Look at the documentation manuals that accompany the software. They should include well-delineated indexes or tables of contents. They should be written in a clear, comprehensible style, that is reasonably free of computer jargon. Staff members will assuredly have questions as they begin to use the system; the manual is the first source for answers.

Once the system is in operation, what sort of "hot-line" telephone support is provided, and at what cost? Is there a mechanism for offering suggestions for program improvements to the vendor? Is the program improved and up-dated periodically? How much will up-date versions cost?

7. Accommodation for Growth

The fund-raising system you purchase should meet your current needs, and be capable of expanding as your development operations grow. If, for example, the system is vendor-installed on a 20 Megabyte hard disk, the vendor should offer some arrangement for re-installing your system on a larger disk when that becomes necessary.

Find out the potential size restrictions of the software itself. If prospect and donor lists double in size, how will the system accommodate that growth? It is reasonable to require that the system be flexible enough to accommodate your operation's anticipated expansion.

CONCLUSION

Because of economic pressures on the private non-profit sector, fund-raising has moved into an era of change and increased requirements for productivity and sophistication. In the micro-computer arena, "change" is also dizzyingly rapid. It is difficult to predict the environment in which one will be working, ten or even five years in the future. Nonetheless, computer systems can so enhance one's fund-raising efforts that many organizations must consider selecting a system now.

A computer system cannot perform the essential creative tasks associated with development work. It cannot describe client services, project an atmosphere of the concern and ethical standards that characterize a social service organization, or produce plans for change that will find community support. This is the task of those who understand and have the skills to work effectively with the community, which many Social Workers clearly do.

However, computer based fundraising systems can help deliver the message to those who believe in the mission of the organization and will support its work. Choosing and implementing the most effective system will require time and effort. A good system will enhance an organization's successful adaptation to a changing economic environment, that shows all signs of placing increasing demands on private fund-raising.

REFERENCES

Abramson, Alan J., and Salamon, Lester M., (1986). *Nonprofits and the New Federal Budget*. Washington, D.C.: The Nonprofit Sector Project, The Urban Institute.

Non-Profit Software Package Review, (1985, Sept.). *Fund-Raising management* 16(7), 74-84.

Meyer, Dennis, (1985, April). Cultivating Major Donors as Greatest Untapped Source. *Fund Raising Management* 16(2), 64-67.

Loykovich, Joan, (1985, Jan.). Special Events in the '80s: A Case for a Marketing Approach. *Fund Raising Management* 15(11), 26-35.

Katz, Wendy, (1985, April). Analysis and Testing of Acquisition Mailings. *Fund Raising Management* 16(2) 52-53.

Sanders, Ralph W., (1985, April). The Donor Profile Survey: A Way to Determine Priorities. *Fund Raising Management* 16(2), 18-27.

BIBLIOGRAPHY

Douglas, James, (1983). *Why Charity?* Beverly Hills, CA: Sage Publications.
Palmer, J.L., and Sawhill, I.V., (eds) (1984). *The Reagan Record*. Washington, D.C.: The Urban Institute Press.

Using Online Databases to Guide Practice and Research

Leonard Gibbs

KEYWORDS. Human services literature, online literature searching, meta-analysis, study synthesis, synthesizing evaluation research

SUMMARY. As tools for human service practitioners and researchers, online databases to locate evaluation literature are becoming increasingly useful. This article uses a clinical problem (concern about the effectiveness of electroconvulsive shock therapy for depressed persons), and a researcher's problem (planning a study to evaluate group treatment for child abusers), to illustrate logic of online searches for evaluation literature. New techniques for synthesizing many studies may require sweeping changes in how abstracts are formulated for bibliographic databases. Study synthesis techniques suggest ways to code studies to describe treatment method, client type, outcome measures, indices of study quality, and indices of treatment effect size. By replacing abstracts with such coded information, evaluation studies could be synthesized continuously for their program and policy implications.

Because human service clinicians and researchers encounter some of the most knotty, complex, and resistive problems faced by

Leonard Gibbs was educated at the University of Wisconsin-Madison, BS (1966), MSW (1968), and PhD (1977). He is currently a Professor of Social Work at the University of Wisconsin-Eau Claire, Eau Claire, WI 54701, and has taught there for nine years. He has published in the following areas: evaluations of juvenile delinquency and alcoholism treatment programs, predicting child abuse, using computers in clinical decision-making, ethical issues in evaluation research, and teaching scientific thinking.

The author wishes to acknowledge support from the University of Wisconsin-Eau Claire Foundation; Carol Kane, Carol Modl, Donna Raleigh, and Diana Sigler for her editorial help.

humankind, they need evidence that is up-to-date, credible, specific to particular problems and in interpretable form. For example, a human service clinician may encounter in a single working week these kinds of problems: child abuse, foster home placement, malnutrition, incompetence due to senility, family disorganization, and drug abuse. Within each of these problem areas questions arise about how to assess risks and how to select the most appropriate intervention, given client characteristics and other factors. Thus, human service clinicians could benefit greatly from a way to locate strong evidence quickly and efficiently.

The human service researcher's needs for evidence are widely known. Researchers who have not taken advantage of online literature searches may want to explore them to save valuable time, to locate up-to-date and appropriate studies, and to locate fellow researchers who have similar interests.

ADVANTAGES OF ONLINE
BIBLIOGRAPHIC DATABASES

Those who use online databases sit at a terminal, or microcomputer that serves as a terminal, to contact, through phone lines, a database kept in the memory of a distant computer. Once the contact is completed, the user makes an identification and applies commands from the database manual to retrieve citations and abstracts that are specific to a particular question.

Databases are especially useful to clinicians who subscribe to the eclectic approach to practice (Fischer, 1978). Since databases do not generally draw a line at discipline boundaries, databases match the needs of eclectic practitioners who may specify type of client, setting, intervention, and demographic characteristics of clients, as descriptors for a search. In addition to being faster than conventional hand search methods — though not necessarily finding better evidence (Gibbs & Johnson, 1984) — some online databases can be used to specify levels of evidence. For example, a searcher might enter the descriptors "random assignment," "randomly," "control groups," to limit a search. A searcher may also retrieve only the most recent studies by searching to a particular date.

SELECTING A DATABASE

Selecting a database should begin with specific questions. Good questions are single barreled (not two or more questions posed as one), are based on a clear understanding of each principal term in the question, and specify at least who, what, where, and when. For example, one might ask, "For parents who become members of Parents Anonymous in the Cook County, what proportion of children are reabused during the two years after the parents join the group, compared with the proportion where similar parents did not join?" Of course, one would need to define: "parents," "membership in Parents Anonymous," "similar," and "reabuse."

Ideally, when such questions arise, one should be able to go to a reference librarian in a large library and have the searches done. But there are also good reasons for conducting one's own searches. Those who need frequent access may find waiting an inconvenience. Some may find it difficult to communicate technical aspects of a search to a librarian, even though the searcher and the librarian have worked together to select descriptors for a search from a thesaurus or database manual. In such cases there is a good chance that a librarian may miss an ideal reference.

Often, one may want to do one's own searches because the local library doesn't subscribe to a particularly appropriate database. There are more than three thousand databases available, and there are about five hundred online services providing access to databases (Directory of Online Databases, 1986). Many databases provide citations and abstracts; some even provide full text. Table 1 lists some example bibliographic databases under the heading "Social Service" from the Directory (1986).

SEARCH LOGIC

I have chosen BRSs Social Work Abstracts (SWAB) to illustrate an online database search. SWAB contains abstracts of over 150 Social Work and other journals as well as doctoral dissertations. Since 1977, approximately 1300 documents have been placed in the database, and over 500 records are added quarterly. Topics covered include: aging, alcoholism and drug abuse, crime and delinquency, economic security, employment, family and child welfare, health

TABLE 1. Bibliographic Databases Listed Under "Social Services" in the Directory of Online Databases*

TOPIC	VENDOR	DESCRIPTION
Child Abuse and Neglect	DIALOG Information Service	Contains citations, with abstracts to materials concerned with the definition, identification, prevention, and treatment of child abuse and neglect.
DHSS-Data	DATA-STAR; Scicon Limited	Contains approximately 50,000 citations, some with abstracts, to the holdings of the DHSS Library concerning health services, social welfare, and social security.
Family Resources	BRS; DIALOG Information Services - Executive Telecom System	Provides more than 80,000 citations covering literature and other resources on marriage and the family.
HDOK	The Swedish Institute for the Handicapped	Contains approximately 2,500 citations to reports on aids for disabled persons.
Social Planning	BRS; DIALOG Information Services	Contains about 8,000 citations, with abstracts, to articles from over 1,200 journals and serials covering the social sciences including social welfare, planning and policy development as applied to specific situations.

*Wordings for these descriptions came directly from the Directory.

and medical care, housing and urban development, mental health, mental retardation, and schools. Other topics in the SWAB database include: social policy, social work methods, social work professional issues, and knowledge from economics, psychiatry, psychology, and sociology.

The basic logic for a SWAB search is similar to that in other bibliographic databases. Generally, once a clear question has been formulated, the user locates appropriate descriptors to specify key concepts in the question. SWAB's descriptors appear in the back of *Social Work Research and Abstracts*. Each descriptor designates a separate set of documents. For example, there may be 100 articles whose abstracts contain the word "schizophrenia" somewhere in the title or abstract. Search strategy concerns basic rules for combining such sets to narrow a search topic.

There are three basic commands most commonly used in searches: "and," "not," and "or." The "and" command indicates that all articles linked with the "and" will be acceptable, that is, a "hit" for the searcher. For example, a researcher may be planning a study of group treatment for child abusers. Here the descriptors would be "group" and "treatment" and "child abusers." Figure 1 below shows the relationship between the three descriptors in an actual SWAB search. The largest circle represents the descriptor with the most hits in the search (N = 3,397). There were also 2,262 hits for "treatment" and another 300 hits for "child abuse" or "child abusers." The intersect between these three circles shows how dramatically the search has been narrowed to 22 hits concerning all three subjects. If the user wants these 22 references, they can be printed later from the disk or while the search is in progress.

The "not" command indicates that any article designated by the first descriptor is a hit, unless that article also contains the second descriptor. For example, the searcher might be interested in "euthanasia," but not in euthanasia for "old age." Figure 2 shows how an actual search for "euthanasia" but *NOT* "old age" found 109 documents for "old age," 6 documents for "euthanasia," and 5 documents for "euthanasia" but not for "old age."

The "or" command indicates that any articles linked with the "or" will be a hit. For example, the term "online" has been spelled "online," "on-line," and "on line." To search for any one

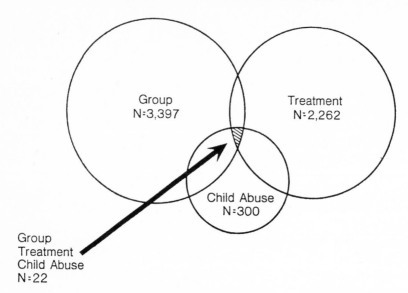

FIGURE 1. The Intersect Between "Group" and "Treatment" and "Child Abuse"

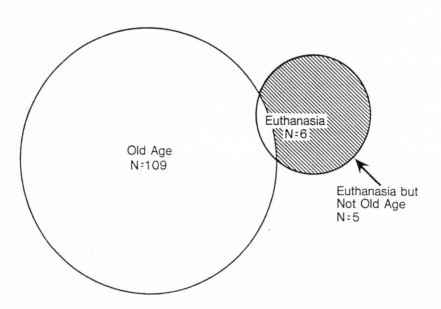

FIGURE 2. A Search for "Euthanasia" but Not for "Old Age"

of these three spellings we can command the computer to search the first "or" the second "or" the third term, thus getting a hit ̲ ̲. any one. In reality, the SWAB search for any one of these three terms found no hits in the SWAB database.

The reader can find more information on bibliographic search strategy in manuals on the subject (Hartner, 1981; Meadow & Cochrane, 1981). Such manuals describe the "and," "not," and "or" commands and more complex uses of Boolean Logic. Boolean Logic is universal for bibliographic database searching. The next section illustrates use of commands in the text of an actual search.

ONE EXAMPLE SEARCH IN THE SWAB DATABASE

Let's assume that a human service worker questions a colleague's recommendation that electroconvulsive shock therapy be used to treat a depressed client who is being counseled at the worker's office. The clinician recoils at the thought of referring a client to a facility where electroconvulsive shock therapy is used, but still the clinician thinks, "Perhaps my objections are unfounded. What is known about the effectiveness of electroconvulsive shock therapy for depressed clients?"

A clinician who has access to the SWAB database can get vital assistance with this life-affecting question. The SWAB search below shows an example search for descriptors: "depression," and "electroconvulsive." The actual text of the search is given on the left of the page below, and the explanation for terms in the search is given on the right. Text that is not essential to the search has been omitted to save space.

TEXT OF A SWAB SEARCH

Computer Printout   Author's Explanation

type CP-6 to access Honeywell CP-6
type PDP to access PDP 11/44
type VAX to access VAX 750

ENTER CLASS rixon
type cr cr to begin
GO

At this point, the system indicates that it is ready to go and the command "rixon" is entered to activate the modem in our system.

RIXON R212A INTELLIGENT
MODEM REV 2
1200 BP

H FOR HELP

$ k
NUMBER: 8369295

The telenet phone number is entered into the computer.

DIALING 8369295
END = !
ON LINE

TELENET
612 13B

TERMINAL =

@c 31520br

User enters the code for the type of terminal being used.

315 20B CONNECTED

At this point, the connection between the vendor's computer and the user's microcomputer is complete.

ENTER BRS PASSWORD
XXXXXXXXX
ENTER SECURITY PASSWORD
XXXXXXXXXXXX
*SIGN ON 21:56:12 10/30/86

These passwords identify the user so no unauthorized person can use the account.

Time and date the search began.

WELCOME TO BRS/BRKTHRU

PLEASE TYPE IN HORIZONTAL LINE LENGTH (20, 40, OR 80).

XX ◆ 80

This tells the computer that the microcomputer can handle 80 characters on each line.

IF YOU ARE USING A VIDEO DISPLAY SCREEN, TYPE IN THE NUMBER OF VERTICAL LINES AVAILABLE ON YOUR SCREEN
XX ◆ 24

The microcomputer's screen can handle 24 lines of text.

THE FOLLOWING SERVICES ARE AVAILABLE:

NUMBER	SERVICE
1	LOOKING FOR INFORMATION?....
2	WANT TO HEAR THE LATEST?....
96	WANT THE LATEST ON THE FINANCIAL SERVICES INDUSTRY?....
97	WANT TO ORDER COPIES OF DOCUMENTS?....
98	WANT TO CHANGE YOUR SECURITY PASSWORD?....
99	SIGN OFF

TYPE IN NUMBER FOR DESIRED SERVICE THEN PRESS ENTER.
XX ◆1

The user's "1" indicates the intent to search for information.

(A LIST OF SUBJECT AREAS AND TYPES OF DATABASES ARE LEFT OUT HERE)

LABEL FOR DATABASE DESIRED
XX ◆swab

The user selects the SWAB database from those listed.

WOULD YOU LIKE DETAILED INSTRUCTIONS THROUGHOUT YOUR SEARCH?
PLEASE TYPE Y OR NO.

XX ◗n

Less-experienced users can ask for detailed, but helpful, instructions for doing their search

WOULD YOU LIKE TO SEE A DE-
SCRIPTION OF THIS DATABASE?
TYPE Y OR N.
XX ◗n

SEARCH TERMS
S1 ◗DEPRESSION

"Depression" is the first descriptor in the search.

A1 354 DOCUMENTS FOUND
SEARCH TERMS
S2 ◗ELECTROCONVULSIVE

There are 354 documents concerning "depression." This is the second descriptor.

A2 DOCUMENTS FOUND

There are 2 documents concerning "electroconvulsive."

SEARCH TERMS
S3 ◗1 and 2

This specifies a search for depression *and* electroconvulsive.

A3 2 DOCUMENTS FOUND

Two documents concern both "electroconvulsive" and "depression."

SEARCH TERMS
S4 ◗d

This option asks to print the documents on the user's computer screen and storage disk for printing later.

SEARCH ANSWER NUMBER
XX ◗3

The text of the search that concerns "S3◗1 and 2" above indicates a particular combination of documents. Here the user has specified that the computer select a set of 2 documents that concern both "electroconvulsive" and "depression."

ENTER S, M, OR L
XX ♦L

The BRS' User's Manual allows the user to specify the amount of material to be printed for each document. The S option merely gives the citation; the M gives citation and descriptors; the L gives detailed descriptions of the articles.

ENTER DOCUMENT NUMBER(S)
OR RANGE OF NUMBERS XX♦1

The searcher indicates only the first document of the two hits should be printed.

One of the two citations from the search regarding electroconvulsive therapy for depressed persons appears below. The headings in capital letters to the left of the citation identify fields in the citation. The OConnell abstract format is typical of those retrieved through bibliographic databases.

AN ACCESSION NUMBER: 11810.
   853.
AU AUTHOR/S: *OConnell-R-A.
TI TITLE: A review of the use of
   electroconvulsive therapy.
SO SOURCE: Hospital and Community Psychiatry, 33(6) : 469-73.
   1982.
AD ADDRESS: *St. Vincent's Hospital and Medical Center, New York, N.Y.
HC HARDCOPY: 21(1), 1985, No.
   376.
DE DESCRIPTOR/S: Electroconvulsive-therapy: review of use of.

This is a citation for a review regarding electroconvulsive therapy.

This is the author's location, should the user want to make contact.

CC CLASSIFICATION CODE:
PSYCHIATRY-AND-MEDICINE
(CC7015).
PT PUBLICATION TYPE:
JOURNAL (J).

AB ABSTRACT: Electroconvulsive therapy (ECT) is an effective psychiatric treatment for severe depression, mania, catatonic states, and, to a lesser degree, some schizophrenias. Complications are minimal and the risk of death extremely low, lower than that for an inadequately treated depression. However, because of advances in psychopharmacology in the late 1950s and the 1960s, some medical centers no longer use ECT. The neurochemical mechanisms that underlie ECT remain unknown, but a cerebral seizure is essential. The average number of treatments is seven, spread over two to three weeks. All candidates for ECT should undergo a complete medical evaluation and give informed consent. (Journal abstract, edited. Nancy Boyd Webb)

This is the abstractor's summary of the article.

LIMITATIONS OF ABSTRACTS

The O'Connell abstract above reveals common problems with abstracts retrieved through databases. First, abstracts can be misleading to a clinician trying to use them. When I located and read O'Connell's original article, my interpretation of the article did not reflect initial impressions based on the abstract. The abstract begins with the assertion that, "Electroconvulsive therapy (ECT) is an effective psychiatric treatment for severe depression, mania, catatonic states, and, to a lesser degree, some schizophrenias." But the article does not review the evidence directly about the effects of ECT. The article's principal focus is on issues regarding how Pto administer ECT including: complications and side effects, procedures for administering ECT, and ethical and legal issues. Surely the abstractor did not intend to mislead me; I simply got the wrong impression from a necessarily brief description.

Second, though O'Connell's review cites references, O'Connell's article does not give enough detail so that I could weigh O'Connell's conclusions for myself. For example, O'Connell mentions several reviews on ECT, cites authors who support ECT's effectiveness, and includes unreferenced impressions: "Studies comparing the effectiveness of ECT with that of antidepressant medications show that ECT is at least as effective." Which studies? How effective against what criteria with what kinds of clients? The review leaves a concerned clinician with too many unanswered questions to make it useful for practical decision making.

The confusion might still remain if, instead of relying on a review, the concerned clinician used references in the database to go directly to original studies that compare ECT against other treatments for depression. Even assuming there were time to locate and read many ECT studies carefully, differences across studies would make cross study comparisons difficult. The studies would vary in their quality; they might show contradictory results, widely different outcome measures, different levels of effectiveness, and might be applied to various types of clients. Making comparisons would be complex and time-consuming. So the vexing problem arises; once abstracts are retrieved, how can we make practical sense of them?

DEFINITION OF META-ANALYSIS
AND AN EXAMPLE

Fortunately, new techniques for synthesizing many evaluation studies are being developed. These techniques are designed to answer practical questions including which treatments are generally most effective, which features of treatment matter most, and which treatments are most effective with particular recipient types (Light, 1984). The appearance of new techniques for data synthesis (Nurius, 1984) or meta-analysis (Glass, 1976) suggest ways to greatly improve present abstract formats. The last part of this chapter outlines how principles of meta-analyses can be applied to improve abstracts in online databases, but first meta-analysis must be defined here.

Glass (1976) first used the term "meta-analysis." To paraphrase Glass, meta-analysis is a statistical analysis of findings from a large number of studies to integrate their findings into a coherent picture. Meta-analysis is a rigorous alternative to a casual, narrative style for reviewing studies that is commonly found in reviews. (O'Connell's review is an example of a narrative one.) Generally, meta-analysis seeks to summarize the effect of treatments in standardized units, rather than relying principally on tests of statistical significance for inferences about treatment effects. By computing an index of effect size in standardized units, meta-analysis gets away from the "voting method" for counting study results based on numbers of studies reporting statistical significance (a finding that favors large sample sizes). Standardized units allow the reviewer to determine the size of an effect for a particular treatment and which treatment is most effective among many treatments.

Since Glass's (1976) pivotal article applying meta-analysis to psychotherapy research, a great deal has been written about meta-analysis. Several books have been written to describe procedures for doing meta-analyses (Glass, McGraw, & Smith, 1981; Light & Pillemer, 1984; Rosenthal, 1984), and reviews on the subject have been written for social service workers (Nurius, 1984). For those who want a quick overview of statistical issues, Hedges (1984) and Wolf (1986) will be useful. Common statistical issues concern the following: how to compute various indices of effect size and significance tests for effect size, how to interpret the magnitude of effect size, and weighting studies by sample size. Others have written about problems with meta-analysis (Strube, Gardner, & Hartmann, 1985; Strube & Hartmann, 1982). Problems commonly referred to in the literature concern: biased selection of studies, reporting inaccuracies, poor quality data, various sources of invalidity and lack of independence for the comparisons reviewed.

In contrast to O'Connell's narrative review, a meta-analysis by Janicak and others (1985), concerning the efficacy of ECT, illustrates typical steps in a meta-analysis and the kind of information needed for meta-analysis. These steps are outlined by Nurius (1984). The first step is clearly defining the purpose of the analysis.

Janicak and his colleagues compared the efficacy of ECT against simulated ECT, placebo, tricyclic drugs, and MAOI drugs in several rigorously controlled studies. Each of these four comparisons is tabled in a section of Janicak's review.

Setting and applying selection criteria is the second step. Janicak and his colleagues did a Medline search of all English-language publications comparing ECT with some other form of treatment for severe depression. Then they narrowed their review to only those studies that met the following criteria: operationally defined depression, random assignment, either double or single blind conditions, and that it could be determined if each subject was a responder or nonresponder to treatment.

Developing a coding scheme for systematically extracting important characteristics of studies is the third step in an analysis. Janicak and his colleagues tabled key features of studies in each of their four comparisons. For each of their four comparisons, Janicak and his colleagues tabled the following: number of treatment responders and nonresponders in ECT, the same proportion for those in each of the four comparison groups, Chi Square and p values for each comparison, the overall difference between the percent improved in ECT compared with that percent in the alternate treatment of placebo group, and a Mantel-Haenszel test statistic (Fleiss, 1981).

Determining and carrying out the statistical analysis most appropriate to the question being studied, is the fourth step. Janicak and his colleagues think previous reviews of studies comparing ECT against other treatments ignored the relatively low power of significance tests reported in their studies. That is, many of the nonsignificant comparisons in previous ECT reviews were based on fewer than 20 subjects. In such comparisons, the chance of finding a falsely negative result (type II error) is extremely high. For example, in the comparison between ECT and tricyclics, three studies reported statistically significant differences, and three did not. The Janicak article uses proportion of responders as its index of effect size.

Interpreting the results and reporting them is the final step. The tables by Janicak and others (1985) show higher efficiency (overall percent of responders) for ECT compared with simulated ECT (32%, p < .001), placebo (41%, p < .001), tricyclics (20% p <

.001), and MAOI drugs (45%, p < .001). The p values reported above are based on chi squares computed by combining study group data according to the Mantel-Haenzel method (Fleiss, 1981).

SUGGESTED FORMAT FOR ABSTRACTS OF EVALUATION STUDIES

Advances in review technology, exemplified in the review by Janicak and others, suggest ways to improve abstracts of evaluation studies. Commonly used abstract format, exemplified in the O'Connell abstract, might be replaced by a tabular format following Janicak's procedure that could facilitate an ongoing integration of evaluation studies. Janicak and his colleagues made 19 comparisons alone between ECT, placebo and other forms of treatment! There are hundreds of questions and thousands of studies that could yield new insights to applications of study synthesis techniques. By using Boolean Logic to locate treatments for particular recipients in particular settings, and abstract formats designed to meet the needs of meta-analysis, it would be possible to do regular ongoing reviews similar to Janicak's for specific clinical and policy decisions. Ongoing analysis that would table effect size, by treatment method, by client type, would require a tabular abstract format for describing key features of evaluation studies.

It may be presumptuous to suggest a format, given space limitations and the early stage of study synthesis techniques, but why not start somewhere? There seem to be three general categories that need specification in abstract fields to make use of study synthesis techniques. The first is study quality. Presently, procedures need to be developed for rating the quality of an evaluation study with measured inter-rater reliability. Many have written about the need to weight study quality in meta-analysis (Bryant & Wortman, 1984; Eysenck, 1978; Kazdin, 1985; Wilson, 1985). There are lists of features of good studies (Davitz & Davitz, 1967; Gehlbach, 1982; Katzer, Cook, & Crouch, 1978) and forms for rating study quality (Chalmers, 1981; Fischer, 1975), but so far no one seems to have measured how reliably a reader can score the quality of a study against a list of weighted criteria. A reliable index should be developed to rate studies. The author is developing one (Gibbs, 1986).

A second field is statistical information. Statistical information should also be tabled in an abstract to aid study synthesis. Here enough should be specified so that reviewers could compute additional indices of effect size if they desired.

A third category should be included in abstracts to help search for recipient-by-treatment interactions. This category should include enough information to identify personal characteristics of recipients in ways that might interact with interventions.

The fields in Table 2 are only suggestions. The information in these three categories could be used to weigh study quality, to compute treatment effect size, and to search for recipient-by-treatment interactions.

Narrative abstracts might be replaced by abstract fields filled in by abstractors who are trained to follow a coding manual. For example, such an abstract might include the usual bibliographic reference and the following coding for *Study Quality*: R_a-yes; R_s-No; C-No; SB-Yes. . . . At first, readers might find such a format confusing, but reader confidence might increase with familiarity. Readers might be able to scan the fields to locate identifying features of subject types, treatment methods, and other information specific to their particular interest. Reader confidence might also increase if abstractors could code study features with measured inter-rater reliability.

CONCLUSIONS

Though not a panacea, online databases are useful tools for practitioners and researchers in human services. Necessitated by the burgeoning evaluation literature, online searches do promise a way to home in on studies that concern particular issues much faster than was possible using old "sniff the abstracts and use the forepaw to retrieve" search methods.

But now a new problem presents itself: how do we make sense of the masses of studies that we retrieve? The next innovations in online databases to human service literature are likely to be sweeping changes in the way studies are abstracted. Abstract formats are now too vague to allow study synthesis. Hopefully, experts in study synthesis will meet with abstractors and database vendors to develop

TABLE 2. Suggested Abstract Fields

Identifying Information

1. Demographics: (Age, Sex, Race, SES)

2. Diagnostic Category (Diagnosis)

3. Diagnostic Procedure (Source for Diagnostic Procedure)

4. Treatment Method (Common name of $T_1, T_2 \ldots T_n$)

Study Quality

1. Random Assignment (R_a)

2. Random Selection (R_s)

3. Non Treated Control (C)

4. Subjects Blind to Treatment (SB)

5. Treaters Blind (TB)

6. Outcome Measured Posttreatment (OUTPOST)

7. Outcome has Inter-Rater Reliability greater than .70 (r)

8. Proportion Entering Treatment to Number at Last Follow-Up (FUP/Enter)

9. Index of Study Quality computed by Adding Weighted Criteria (Stud. Q.)

Statistical Information

1. Number in Treatment Group ($NT_{1,2 \ldots n}$)

2. Standard Deviation of Treatment Group ($SDT_{1,2 \ldots n}$)

3. Number in Control (NC)

4. Standard Deviation of Control (SDC)

5. Mean of Treatment Group –

Mean of Control or Alternate

Treatment Group/Standard

Deviation of Control or

Alternate Treatment Group (ES_1)

6. Proportion of Treatment Responders ($Resp/NT_{1,2 \ldots n}$)

7. Proportion of Treatment Respondees in Control or Alternate Treatment Group (Resp/NC)

8. Test Statistic (Test Stat.)

9. p Value (p)

10. Outcome Measure (Name of Outcome Measure)

Additional Features

Here the abstractor or author could note unique features of each study.

new abstract formats. These new formats may make it possible to monitor the literature regularly to determine which methods are most effective with particular client types against particular outcomes. Regular reports of effect size and study quality regarding particular questions could guide human service workers and policymakers as never before possible.

REFERENCES

BRKTHRU User's Manual. (April 1985). BRS Information Technologies, 1200 Rt. 7, Latham, NY 12110.

Bryant, F. B., & Wortman, P. M. (December 1984). Methodological issues in the meta-analysis of quasi-experiments. In W. H. Yeaton, & P. M. Wortman (Eds.), *Issues in Data Synthesis.* Vol. 24 of New Directions for Program Evaluation, Jossey-Bass: San Francisco.

Chalmers, T. C., Smith, H., Blackburn, B., Silverman, B., Schroeder, B., Reitman, D., & Ambroz, A. (1981). A method for assessing the quality of a randomized control trial. *Controlled Clinical Trials.* 2, 31-49.

Cohen, J. (1977). *Statistical Power Analysis for the Behavioral Sciences.* (Rev. Ed.). New York: Academic Press.

Davitz, J. R., & Davitz, L. L. (1967). *Evaluating Research Proposals in the Behavioral Sciences: A Guide.* (2nd ed.) New York: Teachers College Press.

Directory of Online Databases 7(3). (July 1986). New York: Cuadra/Elsevier.

DRUGINFO and ALCOHOL USE/ABUSE, Drug Information Services, University of Minnesota-Minneapolis, 3-160 Health Sciences Center, Unit F, 308 Harvard St. SE, Minneapolis, MN, 55455.

Eysenck, H. J. (1978). An exercise in mega-silliness. *American Psychologist, 33,* 517.

Fischer, J. (1975). *Analyzing Research: A Guide for Social Workers* (Research Monograph). Honolulu: University of Hawaii, School of Social Work.

Fleiss, J. L. (1981). *Statistical Methods for Rates and Proportions* (2nd ed.), New York: John Wiley & Sons.

Gehlbach, S. H. (1982). *Interpreting the Medical Literature: A Clinician's Guide.* Lexington, MA: D. C. Heath.

Gibbs, L. E., & Johnson, D. (1983). Computer-assisted clinical decision making. *Journal of Social Service Research, 6* (3/4), 119-131.

Gibbs, L. E. (1986). The Quality of Study Rating Form: Teaching fieldwork students to synthesize evaluation studies, Unpublished manuscript, University of Wisconsin-Eau Claire, Eau Claire, Wisconsin.

Glass, G. V., McGraw, B., & Smith, M. L. (1981). *Meta-Analysis in Social Research.* Beverly Hills, CA: Sage.

Glass, G. V. (1976). Primary, Secondary, and Meta-Analysis of Research. *Educational Researcher, 5*(10), 3-8.

Hartner, E. P. (1981). *An Introduction to Automated Literature Searching*. New York: Marcel Dekker.

Hedges, L. V. (1984). Advances in statistical methods for meta-analysis. In W. H. Yeaton & P. M. Wortman (Eds.), *Issues in data synthesis*. Vol. 24 of New Directions for Program Evaluation, Jossey-Bass: San Francisco.

Janicak, P. G., Davis, J. M., Gibbons, R. D., Ericksen, S., Chang, S., & Gallagher, P. (1985). Efficacy of ECT: A meta-analysis. *American Journal of Psychiatry, 142*(3), 297-302.

Katzer, J., Cook, H. H., & Crouch, W. W. (1978). *Evaluating Information: A Guide for Users of Social Science Research*. Reading, MA: Addison-Wesley.

Kazdin, A. E. (1985). The role of meta-analysis in the evaluation of psychotherapy. *Clinical Psychology Review, 5*(1), 49-61.

Light, R. J., & Pillemer, D. B. (1984). *Summing Up: The Science of Reviewing Research*. Cambridge, MA: Harvard University Press.

Light, R. L. (December 1984). Six evaluation issues that synthesis can resolve better than single studies. In W. H. Yeaton, & P. M. Wortman (Eds.), *Issues in Data Synthesis*. Vol. 24 of New Directions for Program Evaluation, Jossey-Bass: San Francisco.

Meadow, C. T., & Cochrane, P. A. (1981). *Basics of Online Searching*. New York: John Wiley & Sons.

Nurius, P. S. (1984). Utility of data synthesis for social work. *Social Work Research and Abstracts, 20*(3), 23-32.

Rosenthal, R. (1984). *Meta-Analytic Procedures for Social Research*. Applied social research methods series (Vol. 6), Beverly Hills, CA: Sage.

Strube, M. J., Gardner, W., & Hartmenn, D. P. (1985). Limitations, liabilities, and obstacles in reviews of the literature: The current status of meta-analysis. *Clinical Psychology Review, 5*(1), 63-78.

Strube, M. J., & Hartmann, D. P. (1982). A critical appraisal of meta-analysis. *British Journal of Clinical Psychology, 21*, 129-139.

Wilson, G. T. (1985). Limitations of meta-analysis in the evaluation of the effects of psychological therapy. *Clinical Psychology Review. 5*(1), 35-47.

Wilson, G. T., & Rachman, S. J. (1983). Meta-analysis and the evaluation of psychotherapy outcomes: Limitations and liabilities. *Journal of Consulting and Clinical Psychology, 51*(1), 54-64.

Wolf, F. M. (1986). *Meta-Analysis: Quantitative Methods for Research Synthesis*. Sage University Series on Quantitative Applications in the Social Sciences, series no. 59. Beverly Hills: Sage.

Statistical Software
in the Human Services:
Old Frontier or Leading Edge?

Richard W. Hug

KEYWORDS. Computers, statistical software, computer literacy, data analysis, human services, professional education

SUMMARY. This article reviews past uses of statistical software in human services organizations and surveys recent developments in the software and its modern substitutes. It proposes four computer literacy standards for human services professionals: (The ability to) (1) choose appropriate software for data analysis tasks, (2) build and analyze small, user-generated data sets, (3) read and analyze external, machine-readable data, and (4) read and analyze internal, machine-readable data. The author concludes that developments in statistical and substitute software have greatly expanded data analysts' options for working with both internal and external data. The developments should help human services pioneers explore both the old frontier of "data rich, information poor" organizations and the new frontier of decision support and expert systems.

There was a time when the "computer person" in a human services agency was the one who knew something about SPSS or one of the other mainframe computer statistical packages. That person, who had learned the skill in a college or graduate school statistics class, used it in the agency to analyze client or employee surveys

Richard W. Hug, PhD, is Assistant Professor of Public and Environmental Affairs and coordinator of the Human Services concentration in the MPA program at Indiana University Northwest, 3400 Broadway, Gary, IN 46408. His research interests include computer applications in the public sector, long term care policy, and the concept of equity in Public Administration.

117

and to prepare reports on service activities and client characteristics in the 40 different formats required by the six different funding sources supporting the agency. It was not always easy work—begging computer time from a local university or cooperating agency, keypunching the data and program, wrangling advice from reluctant programmers, waiting 12 hours to see if the program worked—but it was better than the old way and it was important to be moving the organization into the computer age. Professionals in large human service organizations like welfare departments were beginning to get computer-generated lists of clients, pre-printed forms, and primitive reports but the exciting frontier for human services professionals was the creative use of a mainframe statistical package.

In today's agency, the "computer person" is wordprocessing every memo, letter and report; electronic spreadsheeting every worksheet; electronic filing any useful piece of information in a sophisticated database management system; and telecommunicating whenever possible. Their dreams are of faster and better databases, fancy decision support systems, workable expert systems, and exotic new forms of Artificial Intelligence. But what has become of the old frontier? Is the mainframe statistical package a dinosaur? What about statistical packages for microcomputers? Finally, what, if anything, should human services professionals know about statistical packages in general and what should they be able to do with them?

What follows is a discussion designed to review some tentative answers to the questions posed above. It provides an outline of the knowledge and skill areas considered important for practicing human services professionals. Some notes on suggested resources are appended.

MODERN STATISTICAL SOFTWARE
AND ITS SUBSTITUTES

A case can be made that human services professionals need never bother with mainframe statistical packages. The case rests on two major points: (1) the availability of statistical software for microcomputers and (2) the availability of other software to accomplish the former tasks of mainframe statistical packages.

Scores of statistical packages for microcomputers are now available which advocates contend can do anything that a mainframe package can do and without much of the aggravation. A review of microcomputer statistical packages by Edwin Carpenter (1985) established stringent standards for a "general use" statistical package. Carpenter required his ideal package to handle approximately 200 variables per case and allow virtually unlimited numbers of cases. It had to generate descriptive statistics, perform simple and complex data recodes and transformations, and handle multiple regression, analysis of variance, discriminant analysis, as well as factor and cluster analysis. Carpenter also required log linear analysis, bivariate nominal and ordinal data analysis, and multivariate analysis of variance (p. 184).

In spite of this forbidding list Carpenter found three offerings which managed to meet most of his requirements: two microcomputer versions of mainframe packages, SPSS/PC and BMDPC, and SYSTAT, a package without mainframe ancestry. Since his review, SAS Institute has released a microcomputer version of its highly successful Statistical Analysis System (described below). The fourth major mainframe statistical package, Minitab, also has a microcomputer version. Two important points can be made: (1) microcomputer statistical software is adequate for most research tasks and (2) loyal mainframe users who have been reluctant to learn new software can now keep their familiar language and still enjoy some of the advantages of microcomputers.

Advocates argue that those advantages include convenience, lower costs, control, and, most important for analytical work, graphics capability that is superior to what is available on a mainframe. A microcomputer equipped with a color monitor and a dot matrix printer can create graphs and charts not possible on many mainframes without the addition of special-purpose hardware and software (Hamilton, 1986). Since John Tukey's *Exploratory Data Analysis* (1977), statisticians have become more aware of the importance and utility of graphic displays. For users who are indifferent about the mainframe or microcomputer question, their decision is likely to turn on the need for a strong graphics capability and the equipment and software available on the local mainframe.

The recent availability of superb statistical software and microcomputer advantages in producing graphics are important reasons for arguing that human services professionals need not learn a mainframe statistical package. Just as compelling, however, are the arguments that suggest that there are many substitutes for statistical packages. Chief among the substitutes are database management systems and electronic spreadsheets.

Because they appeared early on the scene, the early versions of mainframe statistical packages were used for many things for which they were not well-suited. The advent of electronic spreadsheets and user-friendly database management systems has gradually retired some of these applications. The latest database management systems allow non-programmers to mimic the COBOL reports of "real" programmers. Before database management systems, human services professionals were forced to make statistical packages accomplish this task. But the packages, which were designed to allow non-programmers to avoid writing FORTRAN programs, turned out to be poor substitutes for accomplishing COBOL-like tasks. Database management systems can produce timely reports of client characteristics and service activities in the formats required by funding agencies. They are more flexible, allow for merging and updating of records and generally simplify the production of the reports that managers need. While they are not capable of producing sophisticated analyses, they have invaded the turf of the statistical packages to the extent that they contain functions for computing counts, sums, means, variances and standard deviations. Some of the more advanced fourth-generation database management systems go so far as to offer optional statistics modules to facilitate analysis.

Electronic spreadsheets have also eased the burden of statistics packages in human services agencies. Spreadsheets (and database management systems) can be used to analyze simple surveys, build and monitor budgets, conduct productivity studies, and perform a host of other tasks which creative users formerly assigned to statistical packages. Like database mangagement systems, spreadsheets are more flexible than statistics packages and generally better-suited to the day-to-day information processing needs of human services professionals. The latest versions of the best spreadsheets have also followed the databases in adding statistical analysis features. While it has always been possible to "program" a first generation spreadsheet to do regression analysis, the latest spreadsheets, offer built-in multiple regression.

A final category of substitute software is a relatively new hybrid which attempts to combine the report and data management capabilities of a database management system with improved data analysis tools. The combination of crosstabulation and graphics capability within a powerful database manager make this type of software attractive for users who want to go beyond simple reports to do the types of things that statistical packages are especially good for. This new type of software, exemplified by Borland International's *Reflex, the Analyst,* is likely to become very popular in the coming years and further erode the domain of standard statistical packages.

But the sellers of mainframe statistical packages have not been content to stand by and let their markets be taken away by the upstart microcomputer software houses. Besides producing their own microcomputer versions, they have worked hard to produce a better mainframe product. By the middle of the 1970s the Statistical Analysis System (SAS) had appeared and begun to challenge SPSS for leadership of the mainframe package group. SAS brought more sophisticated file management capabilities, new statistical procedures, a graphics package, matrix handling capability, report-writing, a more forgiving syntax, and a library of utility procedures. SAS revolutionized computing for research purposes by making it possible for a non-programmer to accomplish sophisticated data processing tasks without having to learn an exotic special-purpose language. Tape handling, reading hierarchical data sets, and merging data from one set to another suddenly became possible for a well-trained research assistant with support from a good programmer. SAS successfully combined a superb set of statistical procedures with a powerful database management system. A student who has learned SPSS in a statistics class can do statistical work. A SAS-trained statistics student understands more about data sets and how they are managed and has a feel for how "real" programmers do their work with computers.

To respond to the SAS challenge, SPSS Inc. produced SPSS-X, a worthy competitor in the statistical package race. Promotional materials for SPSS-X tout it as a productivity enhancer, in the manner of the ads for electronic spreadsheets, databases and the like. The

Table of Contents for their slick, 20-page brochure lists "statistics" only once. File handling, reports and graphs, data management and forecasting sections in the brochure leave little doubt that SPSS is serious about producing a product that accomplishes more than an old-fashioned statistical package.

The makers of Minitab, on the other hand, have not yet produced a product that rivals SAS or SPSS in its data management capability. Minitab's easy to use, interactive, spreadsheet-like program is well-suited for use as a beginning statistical package and for learning about statistics and graphics. Its clumsiness in handling alphabetic data, limits on working with subsets of the data, and its lack of value labels, however, make it less effective as a data analysis tool in human service organizations.

SKILLS

Space limitations preclude a complete discussion of the numerous specific skills required for effective use of statistical software. Instead, the discussion here focuses on three tasks that are proposed as standards for literacy in statistical software for human services professionals (or at least managers, planners, evaluators, and program analysts). Human services professionals should be able to: (1) read, manipulate, and analyze small, user-generated data sets (e.g., employee surveys), (2) read and analyze external data (e.g., a census tape) and (3) locate and/or build and analyze machine-readable internal data sets (e.g., client characteristics).

The planning processes employed in modern human service organizations stress the importance of both internal and external information for strategic decisions (Radford, 1978). But the information required for these decisions and for decisions about everyday operations may not be available in the regularly functioning internal and external information systems. It is sometimes necessary to augment those systems with special analyses of various sorts. For these sorts of tasks, statistical packages are particularly useful.

To say that statistical packages are useful, however, is not to imply that human services organizations most often need the sophisticated modeling capabilities associated with statistical packages. The most useful analysis in most organizations is usually more mundane. Bar charts, histograms, pie charts, scatter plots, averages and simple crosstabulations are often the only displays needed. Analysis, for these situations, involves looking for patterns in the data, checking out hunches, and preparing exhibits that illustrate the patterns and explore the hunches effectively. For this sort of work the vast power of a large statistical package is incidental rather than essential.

For the first task of the literacy standard, reading and analyzing a small data set, this is particularly true. A small, microcomputer-based statistical package serves this purpose well. It is convenient to use and easy to learn because it is menu-driven. It is designed to be transparent — to allow its users to avoid the details of both calculations and difficult syntax in order to focus on the substance of the analysis. As such it can be an important aid in the process of learning how to analyze larger data sets. When a person designs and conducts a survey and has a stake in its outcomes, the desire to explore its results makes preliminary analysis by hand acceptable. That enthusiasm soon drowns, however, in the sea of cross-hatchings, plot points, tick marks, and legends required for a deeper understanding of the data. Using a computer for this sort of project can help insure that the analyst's stamina is not the major factor determining the number of patterns revealed or hunches confirmed or debunked.

When the data set is large, produced elsewhere, and available only in machine-readable form, manual analysis is impossible. The second task, reading and analyzing external data sets, requires a modest extension of the skills needed for the first. In this case the analyst gives up the problems of data entry and verification for a series of other difficulties. Skills needed for this task involve the use of mass storage media: microcomputer diskettes, magnetic tape, and CD-ROM (Compact Disk — Read Only Memory). Under the best of conditions, data made available from other sources may contain errors, be poorly documented, or contain other flaws that challenge the programming and general purpose problem-solving skills of the analyst. In addition, it is important to know where to get data, how to order it in a form compatible with the available hardware and software, and how to transfer it from mainframe to microcomputer and back if necessary.

The U.S. Census Bureau[1] remains as the largest single source of external information likely to be useful to human service organizations. Besides its survey of the population, the Bureau collects and disseminates information about local housing characteristics, state and local expenditures for human services, participation in government income maintenance and other social welfare programs, and data on a host of related matters. Electronic transfer of some Census Bureau data is now a routine process for users of the Bureau's CEN-DATA service.

The Census Bureau is not, however, the only source of external data. Health departments interested in serving pregnant adolescents, for example, can analyze birth certificate data on tapes supplied by a cooperative State Health Department. Birth certificate data can pinpoint the number of births to adolescents and monitor birthweights, Apgar readings, and prenatal care patterns. Such data can provide the geographic detail needed to better target available resources. Human services planners and advocates can compare their state's Medicaid spending patterns over time with that of their neighbors using data supplied on diskettes from the (US) Health Care Financing Administration. National surveys of a wide variety of health services resources are compiled periodically and made available on the Area Resources File, a county level data bank with literally hundreds of demographic and health resource variables.

Sources are also beginning to develop to meet the special data needs of specific types of human service organizations. Colleges and universities, for example, can purchase data on recent high school graduates in their service areas; the degree programs, enrollments, and financial situations of their competitors; and a host of other items destined to become key factors in a marketing plan.[2] Another special source, the Data Archive on Adolescent Pregnancy and Pregnancy Prevention[3] (DAAPPP) recently offered microcomputer or mainframe data on the fee policies of family planning clinics. The newletter containing the announcement also listed 71 other data files of possible interest to program planners and evaluators. For local human services planners the United Way of America has produced a microcomputer database containing almost 100 economic and social indicators for about 300 U.S. communities.[4]

The third and final task proposed for statistical software literacy addresses the perennial problem of professional service in a "data rich, information poor" (Altman, 1976) human service organization. Altman argues that some entities are so busy gathering data that they rarely have time to turn it into useful information. When it is not feasible to enter data for analysis it may be possible to locate or build the appropriate files from the machine-readable data stored by the organization. The skills required for this task are similar to those for task two except that the data are likely to be "dirtier" and the process of obtaining the data more difficult.

The most serious barrier to effective use of statistical software for analysis of internal data is almost certainly the problem of obtaining the required clearances and enlisting programming support for getting the raw data. Stonewalling programmers concerned with their autonomy and prerogatives; overwhelmed managers who feel threatened; clinicians bothered by legitimate confidentiality issues; federal, state and local legal barriers; feuding departments; and assorted other difficulties can result in more time being spent on the preliminaries than on the actual analysis of the data. Successful internal data analysis, therefore, is likely to depend on increased technical capability with the computer in conjunction with more sophisticated ability to satisfy legitimate security concerns and overcome unwarranted resistance.

CONCLUSION/FUTURE DEVELOPMENTS

The microcomputer revolution and the availability of fourth generation computer languages on mainframes have altered the conventional role of statistical software in human service organizations. The concomitant evolution of mainframe statistical software has created an environment in which there are many different ways to accomplish the critical information processing tasks required for survival. These changes suggest important possible developments in (1) professional education and (2) professional practice.

In professional education, modern statistical software has allowed a gradual shift of focus in research and quantitative analysis courses from dealing with calculations to confronting substantive issues in the data. This promise is not new — it was attached to the earliest, most primitive, statistical packages — it is simply coming closer to fulfillment with more user-friendly software. The same software developments have facilitated movement to greater emphasis on exploratory data analysis as opposed to the more traditional confirmatory approach. Both trends lead in the direction of the real goal — better data analysis and research in practice settings.

A caveat is necessary, however. The purchase price of a statistical package does not include training in the appropriate use of the procedures contained therein. Some packages will beep at their users if they attempt calculations that are obviously wrong.[5] Other programs attempt to provide some guidance, but most software and related documentation assume that the user comes to the computer with solid knowledge of the underlying statistical issues (Minor, 1986). Unfortunately, this is often not the case and there are no reliable shortcuts to attaining such knowledge.

A final point on professional education concerns the instructional possibilities raised by the availability of powerful file handling and data management tools within a statistical package. Professional school curricula straining under mandates to increase material on computer applications can use a package like SAS to teach database concepts (Bretschneider, 1986). Or, since fourth generation database management languages (like FOCUS) also include statistical modules, the process can be reversed. In either case, students learn the strengths and purposes of the two types of software without having to learn two different languages.

This discussion began by asking whether statistical packages should be associated with past or with present frontiers of professional practice in the human services. While software substitutes for the early applications of statistical packages are plentiful, a strong case can be made for an expanded and slightly different role for statistical packages in the future.

Human service organizations are still mostly "data rich and information poor." Great opportunities remain for improving practice by turning data into information with the help of a statistical package. Hard-headed analysis using simple techniques on readily available machine-readable data is still relatively rare. Here, the new frontier is much like the old one. It remains as a frontier because it is still poorly mapped and sparsely settled.

For the "new frontier" organization seeking to engage in strategic planning, modern statistical software offers a sophisticated set of tools. Careful analyses of internal and external data, market research, realistic forecasts of future revenues, and effective communication of the results of such work are hallmarks of this organization. For these tasks, statistical software with its associated graphics capability is unsurpassed.

Finally, a cursory review of the literature suggests that the promise of the exotic software of the future rests squarely on the shoulders of work that is likely to be accomplished (if at all) only with strong support from statistical software. Carlson's (1985) list of elements to be included in a clinical decision support system contains an item that requires research on the effectiveness of various treatments for certain types of clients. Vogel (1985) echoes this view and argues that productive uses of decision support systems are unlikely before this research is completed. It appears certain, therefore, that the pioneers of the decision support frontier will have to be armed with some of the refurbished weapons of the previous age. Statistical software, in some form or another, will remain in the survival kit of the modern human services pioneer.

NOTES

1. The Census Bureau's free *Monthly Product Announcement* provides information about new and old products. It is available from the Data User Services Division, Customer Services, Bureau of the Census, Washington, DC 20233.

2. Diskettes of data on higher education are available for sale by National Data Service, 2400 Central Avenue, Suite B-2, Boulder, CO 80301.

3. Tapes and diskettes are available for sale from DAAPPP at Sociometrics Corporation, 3191 Cowper Street, Palo Alto, CA 94306.

4. The package, called Main Street, is available from the United Way of America, 701 North Fairfax Street, Alexandria, VA 22314.

5. Other packages simply refuse to perform. One of my students could not get a package to print a simple table because of "inadequate" cell sizes. This is fine for learning hypothesis testing but not for doing exploratory work with survey data.

6. *PC Week* is published weekly by Ziff-Davis Publishing Co., One Park Avenue, 4th Floor, New York, NY 10016.

7. *SSMR* is published quarterly by Duke University Press, Periodicals Department, 6697 College Station, Durham, NC 27708.

8. ICPSR can be reached at the Institute for Social Research, P.O. Box 1248, Ann Arbor, MI 48106.

9. *U.S. Statistics* is published monthly by U.S. Statistics, P.O. Box 816, Alexandria, VA 22313.
10. See note 1.

REFERENCES

Altman, S. M. (1976). The dilemma of data rich, information poor public service organizations: Analyzing operational data. *Urban Analysis*, 3, 61-75.

BMDP Biomedical Computer Programs: P-Series 1979 (1979). Berkeley, CA: University of California Press.

Bretschneider, S. (1986). Database theory — Lecture 8. In *Summer institute in computer-based instruction for public management, August 4-8, 1986*. Sponsored by the Technology and Information Policy Program, The Maxwell School of Citizenship and Public Affairs, Syracuse University, and The Andrew W. Mellon Foundation.

Carlson, R. W. (1985). Connecting clinical information processing with computer support. *Computers in Human Services*, 1, 51-66.

Carpenter, E. H. (1985). Statistical packages for microcomputers: New visits for social science researchers in 1985. *Social Science Microcomputer Review*, 3, 183-204.

Carpenter, J., Deloria, D., & Morganstein, D. (1984). Statistical software for microcomputers: A comparative analysis of 24 packages. *Byte*, April, 234-264.

Garson, G. D. (1986). *Academic Microcomputing*. Beverly Hills, CA: Sage Publications.

Hamilton, L. C. (1986). Microcomputer graphics for statistical analysis. *Social Science Microcomputer Review*, 4, 181-193.

Kuhlman, J. R. & Lee, E. S. (1986). Data-power to the people. *American Libraries*, 17, 757-760, 778.

Madron, T. W., Tate, C. N., & Brookshire, R. G. (1985). *Using microcomputers in research*. Beverly Hills, CA: Sage Publications.

Miller, D. C. (1986). Running with CD-ROM. *American Libraries*, 17, 754-756.

Minor, M. (1986). Packages can add to market understanding. *PC Week*, November 18, 1986, 194-195.

Monette, D. R., Sullivan, T. J., & DeJong, C. R. (1986). *Applied social research: Tool for the human services*. New York: Holt, Rinehart and Winston.

Radford, K. J. (1978). *Information systems for strategic decisions*. Reston, VA: Reston Publishing Co.

Ryan, T. A., Joiner, B. L., & Ryan, B. F. (1981). *MINITAB Reference Manual*. University Park, PA: Minitab Project, Statistics Department, Pennsylvania State University.

SAS User's Guide, 1979 Edition (1979). Cary, NC: SAS Institute, Inc.

SPSS, Inc. (1984). *SPSS-X Processing of U.S. Census Data*. Chicago: SPSS Inc.

$SPSS^x$: *User's Guide* (1983). New York: McGraw-Hill.

Schrodt, P. A. (1984). *Microcomputer methods for social scientists*. Beverly Hills, CA: Sage Publications.

Tolbert, C. M. (1985). Introduction to computing: Applications for the social sciences. Reading, MA: Addison-Wesley.

Tukey, J. W. (1977). *Exploratory data analysis*. Reading, MA: Addison-Wesley.

Vogel, L. H. (1985). Decision support systems in the human services: Discovering limits to a promising technology. *Computers in Human Services*, 1, 67-80.

Welch, S. & Comer, J. C. (1983). Quantitative methods for Public Administration. Homewood, IL: The Dorsey Press.

APPENDIX: RESOURCES

For a detailed treatment of a variety of issues related to using statistical packages on both microcomputers and mainframes see Tolbert (1985). Less comprehensive coverage can be found in Monette, Sullivan, and DeJong (1986), Schrodt (1984), Garson (1986), or Madron, Tate, and Brookshire (1985). Because of recent rapid changes in microcomputer hardware and statistical software, however, it is important to supplement these general sources with information from current periodicals. For those with little time to monitor such developments in *PC Week*[6] or other such publications, one of the best alternatives is the "News and Notes" section of the *Social Science Microcomputer Review*[7] (SSMR). Besides its coverage of hardware and software developments SSMR includes news of the availability of data in the social science fields which support improved human services practice.

For guidance in selecting microcomputer statistical software and the appropriate hardware see Carpenter, Deloria, and Morganstein (1985), Carpenter (1985), Schrodt (1984) or recent issues of microcomputer periodicals. The April 16, 1986 issue of *PC Week* contains an example of this type of article. A few tips are in order here, though. Welch and Comer (1983) suggest that the ability to produce variable and value labels on printed output is important. Schrodt (1984) warns that crosstabulation is the Achilles heel of microcomputer software. Because of the nature of their data and the types of analyses required, such considerations are critical for human services professionals. Also important is the ability to read data in standard microcomputer formats (e.g., d-Base and Lotus 1-2-3 files) and files transferred from mainframes. For guidance in selecting a mainframe statistical package see Tolbert (1985), *SAS User's Guide, 1979 Edition* (1979), *SPSS[x]: User's Guide* (1983), Ryan, Joiner, and Ryan (1981), and *BMDP Biomedical Computer Programs: P-Series 1979* (1979).

Tolbert (1985) provides a readable chapter on the use of large data sets including some specific information on the characteristics of magnetic tape. The Inter-University Consortium for Political and Social Research[8] (ICPSR) distributes large data sets of interest to human services professionals. U.S. Statistics, Inc.[9] and the U.S. Census Bureau[10] are two other useful sources of information about external data in machine-readable form. A special guide for processing census data using SPSS-X is available from SPSS, Inc. (1984).

For information on the implications of the latest developments in CD-ROM (compact disk—read only memory) technology for mass storage and use of data see Kuhlman and Lee (1986) and Miller (1986). Kuhlman and Lee point out that a single compact disk can accomodate the data on 1500 microcomputer diskettes or four reels of high density magnetic tape. The marketing of relatively inexpensive CD-ROM-to-microcomputer interfaces makes it likely that this new technology will play an important role in human services professionals' plans to analyze machine-readable external data.

SECTION III:
SOFTWARE CREATED BY AND FOR
HUMAN SERVICE PROFESSIONALS

Introduction

The barriers between technology and practice in the human services have been in place for a long time. Service, by its very nature, tends to emphasize the use of self rather than machines or outside materials. Thus, the bridge between technology and service has often been seen as a narrow one — narrow enough to frequently inhibit technology from crossing.

However, in the quest for improved problem solving powers, many human service professionals see a reason for introducing the power of the computer into the realm of service. That reason is the desire to better control and apply the massive amount of information generated in the helping professions. This reasoning has included many possibilities for data input and analysis, up to and including the concept of "storing" the knowledge and experience of professionals in "responsive" programs for use in decision making.

While these concepts and experiences begin to weaken the barriers, the process continues to be a very cautious one. In the forefront of the minds of many is the danger of allowing computer experts to design or manage the information technologies that directly affect service delivery. No means could be more effective in managing

131

this concern – given the invasive potential of the technology – than for human service professionals to take active leadership in the development and use of this software.

Therefore, this section provides examples of the design and introduction of software targeted directly at improving service delivery and its management. The reader will notice that the authors do not attempt to instruct us on the creation process, but instead describe the problem environment that inspired the creativity and the problem solving experience in the development of the software.

As can be seen, the role of the human service professional in software development, especially in the use of assembly or higher level programming language, will normally be as a partner with or as an executive producer for the computer specialists who actually map the software's internal structure and write the requisite code. For this reason, the most successful collaborations of this kind will occur when the human service professional is highly proficient both in the pertinent field of practice and in the use of computers.

A Computer-Integrated Approach to Program Evaluation: A Practical Application Within Residential Services

Melvyn Raider
David Moxley

KEYWORDS. Program evaluation, computerized, information system automation, clinical and direct services, residential treatment, treatment goals and objectives, utilization of evaluation, continuous evaluation process, system specifications, data output format, utilization of software, system maintenance, system modification

SUMMARY. Outcome evaluation of group work intervention in residential agencies. Development of a management/clinical information system and related computer applications.

Program evaluation as discussed in this article describes a service delivery-focused approach to program evaluation which is actually designed and implemented in a residential treatment agency for delinquent youth. The evaluation approach represents a practical strat-

Dr. Raider is Associate Professor of Social Work at Wayne State University, Detroit, MI. He is Chair of the Administration Community Work Concentration in the graduate program of the School. He has consulted with many human service organizations to implement computer integrated program evaluation systems.

Dr. Moxley is Assistant Professor of Social Work at Wayne State University, Detroit, MI. He is also affiliated with the university's Developmental Disabilities Institute where he holds the position of Coordinator of University Relations. This paper reflects Dr. Moxley's continuing interests in the evaluation of human service programs.

133

egy which applies much of the current thinking and research in the area of user focused evaluation. The approach has been refined by incorporating the product of the authors' experiential learning and pragmatic adaptations which evolved out of field testing the model over several years.

The authors present the overall approach to evaluation and the development of the evaluation model within an agency context. The author's then describe the development of a computer-based system which is designed to serve as both a management information system and a clinical information system. Basic aspects of the computer-based evaluation system are presented. Throughout the article, the authors discuss process-related issues pertaining to the introduction of evaluation to both management and staff and movement toward the implementation of an automated evaluation system.

The purpose of this article is to specify the process utilized by a large, residential treatment agency to develop a comprehensive program evaluation model and integrate this model into a system-wide computerized information system. The process illustrates a practical application of both program evaluation and computer technology.

The computer holds several benefits for strengthening the role of evaluation within residential services and can serve as a means of developing human service practice within such settings. The automation of evaluation data enables direct service workers to expand their information base and to ask more complex questions of this information as compared to information which is manually processed. Through the use of the computer, direct service workers can process information on complex and qualitative phenomenon which are needed to create indicators of client outcome. Several variables can be combined into aggregate indicators of individual or family functioning, adaptive behavior and social adjustment, and fed into the clinical and direct service decision-making process. The direct service worker, therefore, can become more oriented to the use of empirical data which is easily processed and accessible given the relative speed of computers as compared to manual procedures.

Using computers within residential settings holds another benefit for human service professionals. Computers have the potential to significantly improve the quality of direct services delivered. With more accessible, relevant, and usable information on client progress in the hands of direct service workers, they are better equipped to make decisions about client care and intervention. The computer can facilitate treatment decision-making and the use of outcome data by teams in monitoring and evaluating client impact on a frequent basis. In addition, direct service workers are provided with more recent and timely information with which to make decisions about the relevance of a client's assessment information, the plan of care, and related treatment goals and objectives.

The authors' approach to program evaluation has a number of dimensions for which the value of computerization is obvious. First, the approach is predicated on active involvement of direct service staff in the planning, implementation, and utilization of evaluation. Active staff involvement not only increases commitment to the program evaluation, but also increases the probability that evaluation will be viewed as a tool to help make intervention more effective (Patton, 1982; Rothman, 1980). Second, the approach emphasizes the significant part ongoing evaluation plays in providing valuable information to enhance the agency functions of planning, coordination and control while the evaluation is in progress. Continuous evaluation feedback allows administrators and practitioners to assess the extent to which service delivery goals are being successfully met and resources are being intelligently utilized (Hagerdorn, 1976). Third, the approach strives to maximize the probability that program evaluation results will be used to make decisions which may improve the ways in which services are delivered. This is accomplished by collecting data which answers evaluation questions of interest to, and actually formulated by, practitioners, supervisors, and managers, i.e., the individuals most likely to use the information (Rothman, 1980).

Finally the approach stresses that in order to be a service delivery and management tool, program evaluation should be an institutionalized, continuous process rather than a series of one shot studies. Indicators of efforts in such areas as services provided, clients served and allocation of staff time are identified, and data are regularly collected, monitored and fed back. Furthermore, the program evaluation approach has been incorporated into a total agency computer-integrated management information system (see Dryer, Koroloff, Bellerby, 1982; Cox, 1982; Austin, 1982).

KEY STEPS IN THE SERVICE-DELIVERY FOCUSED EVALUATION APPROACH

Implementation of the evaluation model involves five steps which are briefly discussed below. Steps four and five, which include designing the data collection format and establishing the data feedback format, are particularly salient for determining computer systems specifications.

Step 1: Identification of the Primary User

In the service delivery approach to program evaluation the direct service worker is viewed as the primary user of program evaluation with agency administrators becoming secondary users. To some extent this view requires a different focus of computer system design as compared to an evaluation model which accepts administrators as the primary users. Administrators are clearly accountable to their boards and funding sources for providing the highest quality services at least cost. However, workers are responsible for practicing in ways which achieve treatment goals and for creating desirable changes in their clients.

Step 2: Establishing the Evaluation Team and Procedures

The second step in the implementing service delivery program evaluation involves establishing an evaluation planning and coordination team. Team membership should include at least one individual representing each of the following perspectives: a member who has both formal and informal influence and power to get the job done; members who are motivated to use the data collected to enhance practice; members who will collect the data; and a member who will be responsible for processing the data and preparing reports for use by direct service workers (see Patton, 1978; Rothman, 1980).

At Boysville of Michigan, the largest residential agency for treatment of delinquent youth in Michigan, several direct service staff were included on the evaluation and planning and coordination team. (Boysville employs over 500 staff members who provide treatment services to over 450 youths in more than 10 locations throughout Michigan.) This involvement resulted in an evaluation design that was more relevant to client needs. It has been suggested that ultimately it is the worker who is most knowledgeable about key aspects of service delivery including practice methods and operational goals (Austin, 1982; Cox, 1982).

In addition to establishing an evaluation planning and coordination team, policies and procedures which integrate the evaluation program into the decision-making structures of the agency must be established (Rothman, 1980). Linkages and procedures also help to increase the prospects that evaluation results will be utilized in the program planning process.

Step 3: Achieving Consensus on Evaluation Focus

To realize the benefits of the service delivery focused approach it is necessary for both workers and administrators to agree upon the evaluation questions to be asked, the ways in which data will be collected to answer these questions, and how these questions may be operationalized so as to be measured. Two issues must be resolved in the process: (1) on what treatment goals should the evaluation focus? (2) how can both workers and administrators achieve consensus on the evaluation focus? Further, the actual process of bringing administrators and workers together to determine program goals to be measured should result in further clarification of program goals and, ideally, reduction in the disparity between formal and operative goals.

Step 4: Designing the Data Collection Format

The fourth step in the service delivery focused approach to evaluation is designing and executing data collection. Concern for the service delivery needs of the worker is reflected in the ways in which data collection procedures are designed and selected. As mentioned earlier workers are involved in establishing the evaluation focus by both identifying broad outcome goals of service as well as by identifying a number of more specific indicators of attainment for each outcome goal. At the design stage practitioners are also involved in determining how each indicator is to be measured. This requires worker participation in the selection of standardized data collection instruments to assure that they satisfactorily measure the identified indicators of outcome goals. Workers may also be involved in the development of instruments to measure indicators of outcome for which no standardized instruments are available. This involvement ensures that the program evaluation tools are actually measuring outcomes which workers are trying to achieve in treatment as well as ensuring measurement of the broader program goals.

The ways in which the above takes place in practice may be illustrated by the process actually used at Boysville of Michigan. As discussed earlier, the evaluation program was developed to assess the effectiveness of providing group work services to the families of delinquent youth concurrent with the youth's residence in the agency. Utilizing the nominal group technique, a major treatment goal was agreed upon by the evaluation team: "the family is to be a functional unit during and after placement." This goal was further delineated into the following subgoals or objectives: (1) increase problem-solving skills; (2) increase use of family and community resources; (3) improve family and child relations; and (4) increase parenting skills.

Workers and administrators subsequently concurred that the standardized Olsen and McCubbin F-Copes scale would be an acceptable measure of the first two subgoals and the FACES II scale by the same researchers would be an acceptable measure of the third subgoal. An original "parenting skills scale" was developed to measure the subgoal of increasing parenting skills.

In this process both workers and administrators were satisfied that the scales chosen actually measured treatment outcomes as well as broader program goals. Further, the selection of standardized instruments, with high reliability and validity, controlled for a potentially significant source of bias and substantially increased the credibility of data collected.

Carefully selected and designed instruments have an additional advantage in that they can significantly reduce the assessment phase of treatment. For example, the data provided by the FACES II instrument administered separately to each member of a family unit may provide the practitioner with insight into the differences and similarities in perception of family dynamics by each family member. Access to such information may be useful in treatment planning. Administering such an instrument can then become a facet of client assessment and treatment rather than a chore to satisfy evaluation requirements.

A final design consideration relates to choosing instruments which may be administered in a short period of time. Administering data collection instruments is an add-on to the workload of the practitioner. To the extent that this can be kept to a minimum, resistance to data collection may also be reduced.

Step 5: Establishing Data Feedback Format

The final step in implementing service delivery focused program evaluation in the agency is the establishment of mechanisms for the regular feedback of data collection results to relevant staff. Feedback of data collection results serves multiple purposes. The ability of the worker to use instruments as treatment monitoring tools is dependent upon the availability of immediate and clear feedback. In order to modify treatment effectively the result of administering measurement instruments such as the FACES scale, discussed earlier, must be provided to workers within a few days. Results of measurement are useless for modifying interventions if they are not current. Further, timely feedback increases worker motivation to administer the scales since such feedback serves as a powerful reinforcer.

The service-delivery focused approach to evaluation requires that practitioners receive timely feedback of results in a fashion which is easily understood. Such graphics as trendline or bar charts, showing client and group changes over time, may increase the likelihood that results will be used in decision-making and planning about client services. Timeliness of feedback enables the worker to modify intervention strategies to make treatment more effective and allows administrators to make programmatic decisions which permit services to evolve and develop over time. Finally, regular and timely feedback of data collection information should encourage continued cooperation from administration and workers in ongoing data collection activities.

General Information Needs

The process described above clearly suggests key dimensions of the program evaluation model which in turn must be considered in specifying the computerized information system. In addition, Boysville is required by its funding sources to report a large quantity of program and fiscal data on a routine and regular timetable. Such data include quarterly treatment objectives, length of stay, truancies, type of referral, post placement living situations, and post placement contact with the justice system.

These data must be reported to funding sources but also have the potential of being used by administrators and workers for treatment planning, program planning, program coordination, and organizational control purposes. Each use will usually require a different output format necessitating a software package that is sufficiently flexible to accomplish this task. For example, funding sources require aggregated reports of post placement status of youth terminated from Boysville according to living situation, school status, work status, and police contacts. Administrators may require this same information for program planning and control. They may wish to cross tabulate post placement status with the demographic characteristics of youth, using such variables as age, race, sex, number of adjudications, number of status offenses and marital status of parents. This report may be useful in establishing criteria for admission into the Boysville program. Similarly, workers may wish to know post placements status of youth for each individual client in the program. This information may be useful for assessing the efficacy of alternate treatment plans and interventions. It may also provide impetus for modifying treatment strategies and techniques to improve postdischarge outcomes.

AUTOMATION OF THE SERVICE-DELIVERY FOCUSED EVALUATION APPROACH

Moving from the process of developing an evaluation approach to the institutionalization of this approach requires that staff perceive significant ongoing benefits from the system. Automation of the process can increase the capacity of the evaluation system to deliver these benefits. For example, a computer-based system can reduce the turn around time from the collection of data to the review of reports by staff.

Automation of the service-delivery focused evaluation approach at Boysville involved the operationalization of several key steps of computer system development. These are: (1) creating an organizational structure for system development and implementation; (2) development of system specifications involving the actual computer hardware; (3) planning the flow and processing of clinical and management data from the point of client entry into the agency and proceeding through follow-up; (4) providing relevant output and feedback to staff at each level of the organization; (5) incorporating existing software into the system so that data can be processed into usable information; (6) maintaining the total system; and (7) planning for how the system will be modified in the future. Each one of these steps is discussed below.

Creation of an Organizational Structure

Boysville has created a research department which has the responsibility for the development, maintenance and modification of the evaluation system, reporting functions, and the automated system itself. The department provides the leadership, continuity, and accountability for the effective implementation of the overall system.

The research department as an organizational structure has both centralized and decentralized features. Responsibilities for system development and implementation are lodged with the Director of Research whose core staff of research, programming and data processing personnel design appropriate software and carry out the centralized tasks of data input, verification, and report generation.

The decentralized aspects of the system assure its integration into the agency as a whole. At noncampus service delivery sites, secretarial staff spend a portion of each week entering data into temporary files. Direct care staff serve in data collection roles by responding to structured instruments and assuring that data is collected at the appropriate time. The involvement of direct care staff in data collection extends from the fact that the approach to evaluation focuses directly on evaluating the effectiveness of service delivery activities.

By designing the basic system to have both centralized and decentralized aspects, the bulk of computer operations and data processing is primarily handled by a specialized unit while program personnel secure service delivery data. Thus, there is a well-articulated division of labor within the organization: one providing organizational supports for the collection of service delivery data and the automated processing of this data.

System Specifications

The data processing system undergirding the service delivery-focused approach to evaluation at Boysville involves the use of microcomputers. The microcomputer system has the capacity to process each case that involves up to 13 data capturing forms and 340 variables.

The whole evaluation system can be accommodated by an IBM-XT personal computer although the agency is currently making use of an IBM-AT. The minimum memory requirements involve 20 megabytes of memory which is sufficient to handle the formation of the agency's relational data base.

Graphics capacity is a critical aspect of the system since reports which are generated for line staff involve charts with two dimensions. The minimum hardware requirements for supporting graphics applications are:

1. Color monitor for graphics display.
2. A Number 9 Revolution Graphics Card.
3. A data product color graphics printer. This printer has a wide carriage and operates at a speed of 400 characters per second in correspondence dot matrix mode.

For the generation of statistical information, Boysville makes use of SPSS-PC which requires a minimum of 384K Random Access Memory (RAM). RAM is internal memory in which the computer keeps data that it is working on, including the programs that are in use.

Systematic Data Collection and Processing

The key to a viable computer-integrated evaluation system is the use of structured data capturing instruments. As noted above, the Boysville system makes use of up to 13 data capturing forms which are used by direct care staff at key points in the client pathway: at intake and client entry, during service delivery and intervention for both individual clients and their families, and at the points of discharge and follow-up. The data capturing instruments make use of client self-reports, staff ratings of individual children and families, and checklists.

Data collection requires staff commitment but not an excessive amount of staff time. Staff members are trained to use the instruments when they enter the agency, when an instrument is modified, and when data collection begins to decrease in quality. A user instruction manual containing all instruments and itemized instructions for completing forms is accessible to all line personnel.

Another means of supporting data collection of high quality is an automated "tickler" system. Line staff receive lists of clients who are to be observed and the instruments which must be completed well ahead of the scheduled time of completion. Supervisors also receive ticklers reminding them of the data collection schedule and identifying staff members who must collect the necessary data. A master code book identifies key variables and the values of these variables.

Since all data capturing forms are highly structured, the data entry clerks do not have to make decisions about entry. They enter the data directly into the machine according to screen formats that correspond to the data capturing forms.

Data entry is the responsibility of clerks at the main campus location while at offsite locations secretaries are responsible for data entry. Entry of data is made into a temporary file on a manual basis. Machine verification of the data occurs when the data elements are being entered into the temporary file. The machine will make a sound when a mistake is detected. Typical errors that are detected at point of entry involve out of range values, site number, client name, and client identification number. Once the data is loaded into the temporary file and machine verified, it is electronically transferred to the master data file.

Output and Feedback

System output is numerical and graphic. Reports are generated containing numerical information on client change in key areas of psychosocial functioning, family adjustment, and service provision such as length of stay and resource allocation. Output is summarized in three types of routine reports involving aggregation of data at three levels of the organization:

1. Direct Service Reports. Line workers receive reports of individual clients which show client status and change on relevant psychosocial indices derived from data collection instruments as well as client status and change over time. These reports consist of two-dimensional figures with time reported on the X-Axis and the relevant psychosocial index on the Y-Axis. Graphs showing a client's change is then displayed as a trendline.

2. Program or Unit Reports. Information is aggregated by worker or team and is reported in numerical format usually involving numbers of clients, numbers of contacts and percentages. Information pertaining to client progress and contact levels with families are reported. These reports are designed for training and supervision purposes so that the effectiveness of workers and teams can be monitored on an ongoing basis. When there is indication that contacts are not being made with certain types of families at the desired level or certain children are not making progress, the training department of the agency can focus on specific skill-building or attitudinal areas while supervisors can review specific cases with individual workers or teams.

3. Regional Reports. The third level of routine aggregation occurs at a regional level. These reports serve management information purposes. Numerical information on such variables as terminations, movement through the system and child and family status at various follow-up points is summarized for each regional administrator.

All reports incorporate statistical analyses. Routine statistical information reported to direct service staff usually involves univariate frequencies summarizing clinical data on children under the care of individual staff members. Cross-tabulations of data and other bivariate analyses are incorporated into program and regional reports. Multivariate analyses of clinical and outcome data are usually disseminated to all staff through occasional research bulletins prepared by the research department. These bulletins focus on key service delivery questions or trends and report regression analyses or differences between groups of children based on status or program variables.

Utilization of Software

The software needed to operate the Boysville system incorporates existing software packages and the creation of in-house procedures. The latter have been written by either the agency's Director of Research or by an external programming consultant.

The computer system operates as a menu-driven data base management system. Such programming languages as TURBO PASCAL and DR. HALO were used to design screen and graphic procedures. Screen formats were created by defining data sets, specifying numeric field widths, and by specifying verification edits. Data entry is facilitated by a structured videoscreen format that requires the entry of data of predetermined specifications. SPSS-PC, a statistical package designed for personal computers, is used by the research department for univariate, bivariate, and multivariate analysis of evaluation data.

System Maintenance

The major aspects of system maintenance are intimately connected with its human dimensions. Maintenance is based on staff deriving benefits from the evaluation data and its automation. Timely feedback is routinized thereby assuring the provision of information to staff which is relevant to service delivery decisions. A short turnaround time – that is, the time from staff completion of forms to the generation of reports – is approximately four days.

Assuring the entry of quality information is another vital aspect of system maintenance. At Boysville there is a strong linkage between the research and training departments which enables the agency to maintain a cadre of staff members who are effectively trained in the nuances of data capturing instruments and data collection procedures.

System maintenance is facilitated by the ease with which the system is integrated into the work routines of the agency. The research department serves as a centralized support structure responsible for perpetuating the system. Data collection responsibilities serve both clinical assessment and evaluation purposes. The data collection process takes approximately one day per week for 125 children. This translates into approximately two person days.

Each secretary who manually enters data into the machine does not exceed four hours of data entry work each week. The system, therefore, is not unreasonable in the amount of time required of participants to maintain the flow of evaluative data.

System Modification

Shortrun system change involves the actual expansion and augmentation of the evaluation data base. The agency is reluctant to delete any of the data elements currently being collected. This will assure the development of a strong historical data base which will be useful in monitoring service delivery over time. Staff recognize, however, that new problems are being identified and addressed at Boysville on an ongoing basis. Changes in client problems and needs are being communicated by service delivery staff to the research department which in turn examines the need for the addition to the data base of relevant indicators of these emerging problems and needs. Necessary changes are then made to the data capturing and data collection procedures.

Such a modification was recently made. Child sexual abuse is recognized by staff as a problem among children and families served by the agency. This has resulted in the addition of questions focusing on sexual abuse to the data capturing instruments. Subsequent analysis of these variables reveals that a significant portion of children and families served by the agency are coping with this problem.

Longterm system change will involve the networking of micro-computers and the decentralization of their online use. The agency is looking to the creation of an interactive microcomputer system allowing managers to directly interact with the machine and conduct nonroutine analyses of data based on their own supervisory and program needs.

CONCLUSION

In order to make major inroads into the development and institutionalization of a computer-integrated evaluation approach focused on service delivery, Boysville of Michigan has had to implement two different but complementary processes. One process involves the actual development of the evaluation model. As we have outlined this is very much a collaborative process which requires input and participation from both direct service staff and administration. Another process is the actual development of an automated system for supporting the processing and reporting of evaluative information. This undertaking has been largely centralized at Boysville by virtue of building an organizational structure dedicated to research and evaluation. The success of this automation, however, has involved the decentralization within the agency of some key responsibilities for data collection and processing.

From our perspective, the key to this evaluation approach lies in appreciating the human element of the system. Boysville has not lost sight of the need to design the system so that it accrues benefits for the direct service workers who make use of it. The agency also recognizes the importance of making the maintenance of the system a feasible process. The system needs to be integrated into the actual work structure of the organization, without making inordinate demands on those who are responsible for making it work.

The development of the system and its automation has required the agency to become proficient in all aspects of data processing, data management, software use and design, and the use of micro-computers within a human service environment. This burden has been mainly absorbed by the research department of the agency. As an interactive system is developed and implemented, program administrators will have to become better versed in the use of microcomputers. The actual creation of an effective interactive system and the training of managers to make use of it is the next major step in the evolution of service-delivery focused evaluation at Boysville of Michigan.

REFERENCES

Austin, M. J. (1982). *Evaluating your agency's programs*. Beverly Hills, California: Sage.

Cox, G. B. (1982). Program evaluation. In M. J. Austin and W. E. Hershey (Eds.), *Handbook on mental health administration*. San Francisco: Jossey Bass.

Delbecq, A. L., Van deVen, A. H., and Gustafson, D. H. (1975). *Group techniques for program planning*. Glenview, Illinois: Scott Foresman and Company.

Epstein, I., and Tripodi, T. (1975). *Research techniques for program planning, monitoring and evaluation*. New York: Columbia University Press.

Garvin, C. (1981). *Contemporary group work*. Englewood Cliffs, New Jersey: Prentice-Hall.

Hagedorn, H. J. et al. (1976). *A working manual of simple program evaluation techniques for community mental health centers*. Washington, D. C.: United States Government Printing Office.

Hakel, M. D. et al. (1982). *Making it happen: Designing research with implementation in mind*. Beverly Hills, California: Sage.

Olson, D. H. and McCubbin, F-Copes, FACES II. University of Minnesota, 290 McNeal Hall, St. Paul, Minnesota, 55108.

Patton, M. (1978). *Utilization Focused Evaluation*. Beverly Hills, California: Sage.

Raider, M. (1987). A service delivery focused approach to evaluation in residential treatment agencies. *Residential Treatment for Children and Youth*. 4(3).

Rossi, P. and Williams, W. (1972). *Evaluating social programs: Theory, practice and politics*. New York: Seminar Press.

Rothman, L. (1980). *Using research in organizations*. Beverly Hills, California: Sage.

Rutman, L. (1977). *Evaluation research methods: A basic guide*. Beverly Hills, California: Sage.

Tripodi, T. et al. (1978). *Differential social program evaluation*. Itasca, Illinois: F. E. Peacock.

The Making of COBRS 2.0: The Competency-Oriented Behavior Rating System for Children and Youth Services

George Thomas

KEYWORDS. Children's services, youth services, computerized behavior assessment, computerized program evaluation, behavior assessment theory.

SUMMARY. Recently introduced advances in microcomputer technology offer opportunities for improving child welfare agencies' access to powerful case assessment and program evaluation tools. This paper discusses the process of fitting a child behavior outcome measurement system to a menu driven microcomputer program. Traditional strategies for measuring outcome effectiveness, managerial priorities and operational constraints are examined in terms of their bearing on the introduction of new microcomputer technology. The developmental process is traced to show how these factors influenced the addition of a number of user options to the basic program to enhance its adaptability to specific agency needs. Initial user feedback indicated general satisfaction with the basic program and the applicability of its output, little or no experimentation, as yet, in adapting the system, and, a minor need to adjust the sequencing of operator activities to better fit the realities of agency work rhythms.

Dr. Thomas is President of George Thomas & Associates, Ltd., P.O. Box 152, Athens, GA 30603. Dr. Thomas continues to pursue a career interest in applying state of the art research and development technology to enhance client service and staff development programs in the field of children and youth social services.

149

INTRODUCTION

What follows are observations and comments about the interplay between measurement, management, and computerization issues in the field of group residential child care services that helped shape COBRS 2.0 into its present microcomputer supported form. The simple moral illustrated by this tale is that if evaluation technology in children and youth services is to be advanced by a new application program, its construction must be guided by a firm grasp of the demands and limitations imposed on the state of the art by the interplay of certain issues.

COBRS 2.0 is a competency-oriented child behavior outcome measurement system designed to provide decision support in the conduct of case assessment, program evaluation and staff performance monitoring activities. The system is supported by a microcomputer program compiled from dBASE III that operates on IBM or compatible microcomputers with DOS 2.0 or higher, 320k RAM and 2 disk drives, or a hard disk. Data input is accomplished by use of 5 data entry forms. Two are used to create child and personnel case records, one to enter staff observations of child behavior, and two for obtaining child self reports of behavior. Report output, for program evaluation purposes, includes weekly and quarterly tables and time trend graphs for child behavior profile data grouped by categories of 10 report generating variables. Case assessment is facilitated by weekly tables, time trend graphs and pre/post analyses of behavioral performance/progress for individual cases. Case and personnel file record printouts can be obtained, as needed, for record editing and case tracking purposes.

COBRS 2.0 is completely menu driven and fitted with a wide variety of user options for future growth. Users may define report variables and case tracking variables in setting up their record keeping and report output systems. Further, they may edit item content in all data entry forms to fit differing service settings (residential, in home, etc.) and/or client cultural orientations. Finally, they may set a statistical goal model against which agency specific goal achievement may be measured.

Initially designed for residential group care services for older children and youth, COBRS 2.0 is adaptable for use in follow-up and day treatment services, school classrooms for behaviorally disturbed children, foster family care and independent living programs. Program upgrades are also in process to automate data input by interfacing with desk top optical scanners, to permit multiple site data aggregation and to transfer case data from existing MIS to avoid input duplication in creating case records.

IS THERE A NEED FOR YET ANOTHER CHILD BEHAVIOR OUTCOME MEASUREMENT SYSTEM?

At first blush, the logical answer to this question would seem to be, "no." At least the need is not self-evident in the pertinent post-war history of child welfare services extending through the 70s. This era has been characterized as one of wide-spread developmental activity on the part of agencies and independent researchers that yielded, nonetheless, little in the way of sustained application in practice (Magura & Moses 1986:2ff).

This disparity is perplexing because official agency mission statements are commonly couched in child development rhetoric which would dictate, it might be thought, the use of such a system to meet accountability needs. On reflection, two factors interdict the connection between mission and measurement and lend understanding to the disparity; namely, the nature of public accountability demands and the technical shortcomings of available systems.

1. The Shifting Demand for Outcome Accountability: From Proof of Problem Reduction and Program Compliance to Evidence of Preparation for Life

It is often said that we manage what we measure. It might be added that we measure that which is pertinent to our immediate survival and prosperity. In this regard, the post-war era through the 70s can be roughly divided into two distinctly different periods in terms of accountability demands. First came a time of public acquiescence to professional authority and expertise. There followed a stretch marked by an emphasis on program compliance monitoring which was spurred by a rapid growth in program funding by federal and state agencies.

Early on, professional interests in theories of abnormal behavior, problem-solving practice methods and problem-oriented record keeping held sway. In effect, accountability took on an insular "take my word for it" quality. Consistent with its orientations, the professional establishment set behavior problem reduction goals and then proceeded to determine success in accord with its own standards (Shyne 1959). Later, this approach to accountability was overtaken by a quite different set of governmental priorities intent on obtaining "body count" data, which tended to use the terms "effectiveness" and "compliance" interchangeably (Combs 1979; Mutschler & Hasenfeld 1986). Neither accountability approach required much in the way of child behavior outcome measures, and neither produced much in the way of direct evidence of mission accomplishment; but then, mission fulfillment was not directly linked to accountability and issues of survival.

The 80s have brought about profound changes in public notions of agency accountability. The public's post-Vietnam/Watergate disillusionment with authority and expertise of any kind is reflected, no doubt, in the demands being imposed on agencies by the national child maltreatment prevention movement and the recent surge in malpractice litigation. As Besharov notes, "Social workers no longer enjoy unfettered freedom to do what they claim is in the best interests of children and parents" (Besharov 1985:15).

Professional assertions can no longer be counted upon to satisfy public accountability demands and the practice of substituting program compliance data as proof of effectiveness — a common occurrence in recent years, is also on shaky ground. Nutter, Gripton & Murphy (1986), drawing on their findings from a survey of computer supported information systems in the social services in Canada, pose a telling question for compliance type systems: "Can information which is not adequate as the basis for individual case decisions be adequate for decisions affecting hundreds and thousands of cases?" Although present practices, in their judgment, seem to reflect an implicit yes answer, the authors conclude that, "No is a more sensible answer" (Nutter, Gripton & Murphy 1986:6).

Perhaps of most importance, public attention is swinging toward preventative services that aim to reach children before problems arise and to prepare them in the "soft" and "hard" skills needed to assure their continued acceptable development and transition to independent living (Hamburg 1986, NAFFC Newsletter 1987). Behavioral competency development has taken hold as the critical goal for children and youth services (Maluccio 1981; Ainsworth 1985; Gaylin 1982; Kent & Rolf 1973) and it can be expected that as these influences become more articulated in the public mind, demand for accountability in competency-oriented behavioral development terms will intensify.

2. Technical Shortcomings in Existing Child Behavior Measurement Outcome Systems

Accountability issues aside, it does not make sense to use a child behavior outcome measurement system that does not support a higher proportion of reliable and valid case and program decisions than would otherwise occur. In a general sense, this explains why agencies, often after long years of trial and error exploration in designing and/or adapting such systems, give up on them and revert to staff case conferencing and related decision support methods (Mordock 1986; Thomas 1967).

The extent to which a particular child behavior outcome measurement system falls short of agency needs, particularly in light of emerging accountability demands, can be determined by examining several factors, including: the proportion of the total child behavior domain measured; the clarity with which it is measured; who and how many do the measuring; how often measurement occurs; how easily data are retrieved; and, how broadly output can be applied for decision support purposes.

To begin, features common to many existing child behavior outcome measurement systems limit their usefulness by being manually driven and by focusing narrowly on the problematic part of the total child behavior domain. Additionally, they tend to rely heavily on technical measurement terms (e.g., "negligent fire setting, phobic, eating disorder, sex disturbance, etc.") which necessitate ei-

ther detailed definitions and scoring instructions or the use of extensively trained or professional observers (Magura & Moses 1986:
23-76; Nelson, Singer & Johnson 1978; Wilson & Lyman 1983).

Partly because of limitations imposed by manual operations, data
collection is often limited to the use of a single observer at infrequent intervals (6 weeks or longer). Results are often issued in rudimentary form, mostly as individual case scores and less frequently
as group aggregates. Only very rarely are they expressed in terms of
time trends.

The reliability and validity of practice decisions based on data
produced by systems possessing a few to all of these limitations
tend to suffer. For example, it is illogical to suppose, although the
belief seems wide spread in practice, that accurate predictions about
a whole child's behavior and future prospects can be made from
knowledge about a small part (the problematic part) of his behavior,
no matter how detailed that knowledge is (Hambleton 1985:399). In
practical terms, such extrapolations contain a large margin for error
since they implicitly equate an absence of problem behavior with
general behavioral competency, or normality.

Among the many reasons why this is a faulty assumption is the
fact that problem behaviors are proportionally rare with the context
of the total domain of child behavior, even in therapeutic environments. Thus, when problematic behavior is the central focus for
observations and reporting, errors in judgment can arise simply by
taking what is naturally a relatively infrequent occurrence as evidence of progress.

On the other hand, problematic behavior can be manufactured in
the sense of seeing more than occurs. This can happen when ob-
servers/reporters must attain an intricate and commonly agreed-to
understanding of behavior terms before making observations about
them, leading observers to read meaning into observed behavior to
fit textbook definitions. This is one reason why some child behavior
measurement instruments with high reliabilities, in the traditional
statistical sense, may produce less than meaningful and useful information for making decisions in practice (Krotkotwill, Mace &
Mott 1985:354).

Finally, to the extent that a system depends on single observers
and infrequent observational periods, much behavior that occurs

outside the scope of the observer, or between data collection periods, will obviously go unreported. The reliability and validity hazards here take the shape of what Mordock (1987:70) refers to as a "halo effect," that is, a tendency to generalize currently observed behavior as representative of behavior for the entire period between observations, or from the perspective of one observer as representative of multiple perspectives.

In sum, the various factors that account for a lack of use of child behavior outcome measurement systems in practice contribute to a condition in which many agencies may be achieving more in the way of child development mission accomplishment than they are measuring. In turn, they may be reporting less to their supporting public constituencies than they are, in fact, accomplishing. From all of this, the requirements of a useable system were plucked, bit by piece, and integrated to form COBRS 2.0.

PUTTING IT TOGETHER: MEETING THE REQUIREMENTS FOR A USABLE CHILD BEHAVIOR OUTCOME MEASUREMENT SYSTEM

1. A Unitary Decision Support Data Base for Evaluation at All Levels That Yields Reliable, Valid Data

Measurement/Data Base Requirements. A single "bottom line, bottom up" data base is a critical need. The bottom line is child behavior performance and progress. Such data are directly informative about mission accomplishment and can be used in different aggregates to perform case assessment, program evaluation and staff performance monitoring at various organizational levels. "Bottom up" means collecting data from sources in a position to most accurately report child behavior, namely, adults who share children's daily lives, and children themselves.

In practice, data reliability and validity are closely linked. Data reliability depends on maximizing the correspondence between what is observed and what is reported. Data validity depends on assuring that what is observed is a consistently accurate representation of the domain of child behavior needed to support accurate evaluation decisions.

COBRS 2.0 Response. To meet this requirement, COBRS 2.0 utilizes one adult (BRS) and two child self report (TSRCS & LOC) observation/reporting data entry forms that have been developed and refined over years of field research. Their methods of development and reliability and validity estimates for the data they produce are provided in a following section.

In addition to the quality of the data entry forms, the data collection process has been structured to gather multiple direct observations of child behavior from multiple observers (two adults and the child) at frequent (weekly) intervals to assure the establishment of a consistent and comprehensive representation of the key child behavior domain essential for decision support purposes.

Finally, the software program contains on-screen instructions for operators at every point of data entry, and program safeguards that permit only legitimate numerical values to be entered. These features minimize prospects for data entry errors at the keyboard.

2. Computer Support: Time/Cost Economy in Implementation and Operation

Computer Requirements. There is growing consumer awareness that there is no magic in computerizing anything (Fleit 1987). Agency managers, in particular, tend to express legitimate concerns over the prospects that the introduction of computerized information systems might lead to a loss of internal control due to a continuing dependence on technocratic expertise, and that reduced productivity might result from the need to divert mission related resources to their ongoing care and feeding (Rubin 1976; Rimer 1986). By implication, a usable computerized system had to be operable by staff on hand.

COBRS 2.0 Response. From the outset of software development, COBRS 2.0 was designed to be microcomputer based, completely menu driven and supported by a clear and detailed self-instructional manual covering everything from set-up logistics to guidelines for score interpretations. In short, it requires no outside expertise to set up. And, extensive field testing indicates that, on average, the system requires no more than 10 minutes of staff time, per child, per week, to complete operations from reporting observations to report output. This level of efficiency in operations also suggests little or no need for additional staff.

Secondly, field testing under manual conditions indicates that all of the data entry forms and data collection procedures work well in real-world conditions with minimum staff indoctrination, thereby avoiding the time/cost burdens required by protracted staff training.

Thirdly, the Case Record and Personnel File data entry forms were initially developed, along with the original software program, during a time before such terms as megabyte and hard disk had entered the lexicon of microcomputers. This meant that a kind of data entry economy was built into these forms to accommodate microcomputer memory and disk storage limitations. That economy remains a favorable operational feature in the current, larger program version. To explain, these forms permit user definition and entry of 16 and 19 variables respectively. Coding variables for data entry is performed by applying user-developed hard copy code sheets. In comparative assessments, this approach has proven capable of coding all the information in two currently used presence/absence type behavior problem check lists of 64 and 89 item lengths, respectively, by judiciously using 2 or 3 COBRS 2.0 data entry variables and associated hard copy codes.

Finally, all reported scores, with one exception, are provided in simple two-digit percent form to allow direct interpretation and use of quantitative data by all levels of staff.

3. User Demands: System Adaptability, Evolutionary Change and Wider By-Product Benefits

User requirements. Reports from users of the original 1.2 version of COBRS indicated that they had more agency specific needs and broader perspectives about the impact of computerized information systems than we had envisioned in our design. Some wished to modify all of the 5 data entry forms to enable tracking for case characteristics specific to agency needs. Others saw a need for options in changing item content in reporting instruments to allow measurement of child behavior outcomes better fitted to agency specific service contexts and/or goals. Still others wanted a choice in restructuring the pre-set statistical goal model to fit their own definitions of success in behavioral outcomes. In short, early user feedback suggested that a system without adaptability would have a short life.

It also became clear that administrators preferred the pace of change following introduction of a computerized information system to be evolutionary rather than abrupt. The information thus produced should have a capacity for a broader impact on staff communication and goal clarity, in particular, which could be planned for and gradually achieved. It was acknowledged that abrupt change could bring about just the opposite, on all counts.

COBRS 2.0 Response. Regarding adaptability issues, all COBRS 2.0 data entry routines and the routine governing the structure of the statistical goal model for measuring achievement were transferred from hard code to data bases and the data entry forms were modified to permit users to define/code their own report generation (N = 6) and case tracking (N = 9) variables. These changes also enabled users to apply a self-instructional methodology for empirically constructing and entering their own statistical model for measuring goal achievement. Finally, users would now be permitted to edit the item content on the 3 behavior observation/reporting forms (BRS, TSRCS & LOC) to fit measurement needs in specific service contexts or for clienteles with varying cultural heritages. For example, if services were to be provided in the home context a term like "cottage counselors" in the item, "My cottage counselors yell at me a lot," could be changed to, "parents." This does not alter the meaning of the item but it does better suit it to measurement needs within in-home service settings.

In addition to these features, the pace of implementation is determined in-house. This, combined with effects that can be expected from the infiltration of "bottom line, bottom up" information, assures users that they will be in control and can expect gradual emergence of improved staff communication, goal clarity and better decision-making. To examine how this might work in the real world, it is instructive to review the information structure in a "typical" children and youth group residential care program that has been constructed in composite fashion from a study of 32 such facilities (Thomas 1975).

At the top is a partially computer driven compliance monitoring system that turns out "body count" reports used primarily by management. Positioned in the middle is the problem-oriented child behavior measurement/case assessment system developed and manually operated by professional staff. This system relies on a rich mix of idiosyncratic and technical data lodged in process recordings and frequent exchanges in staff meetings. Copious amounts of time are spent defining terms, negotiating meanings and defending viewpoints in the decision-making process. At the bottom is a sub-rosa manually driven system that circulates masses of direct observations about child behavior among direct service staff that are used simultaneously to manage personal stress and child behavior. In the absence of any better guidelines, personal values are commonly used by direct service staff to interpret these data and to apply them to achieve desired child behavior outcomes. These values may vary considerably from mission intent and produce "institutional adjustment," that is, behavioral conformity to rules and standards contrary to goals for growth and development. This heavy reliance on personal values by direct service staff may encourage the development of incompetent behavior, and worse, responses of an abusive sort when conformity is not forthcoming (Rindfliesch 1984:55).

The "bottom line, bottom up" structure of COBRS 2.0 has its greatest immediate impact on direct service staff by redirecting attention and reporting away from institutional adjustment and toward competency-oriented behavioral performance, and by according these staff an official role in the decision-making process. Both impacts should have clear and favorable upward effects. Gradual change is also the mode expected at the professional and managerial staff levels. Here, roles and functions are not immediately changed, but role performances will be enhanced by information supplied by the system. As the impact of using a more organized, comprehensive, pertinent and reliable data base sinks in, refinements in professional staff decision-making can be expected. And, as managers become accustomed to using direct rather than inferential evidence to evaluate mission accomplishment, efficiency in perceiving and responding to what's going right and what needs to be changed can be expected to improve. In turn, more efficient staff communication and greater goal clarity will likely obtain.

HOW IT ALL WORKS:
FROM CREATING AND INTERPRETING SCORES
TO TYPES OF REPORTS AND THEIR USE

1. The Development of Observation/Reporting Data Entry Forms and Their Scores

The Behavior Rating Scale (BRS)

The BRS is composed of 49 brief behavior statements (e.g., Works well alone, Boasts, Listens to me, etc.) and a 50th space for reporting the number of Critical Incidents (CIs) — or seriously deviant behavior episodes as defined by the user, which are narratively described on the form's reverse side. Each item is scored in terms of its observed frequency (None, Some, A Lot) by two independent observers on separate observation days, each week. Negatively and positively phrased and scored items are intermixed, and are organized under sub-headings that do not correspond to the item clusters for behavior dimensions, to minimize observer response set. Item cluster scores are computed and reported in two-digit percent form ranging from 0 to 100 which together represent a profile of 6 behavior dimension scores, and a total score, as follows:

- Self Discipline   (From undisciplined to self disciplined)
- Exemplary   (From poor to good peer role model)
- Conforming   (From unruly to accepting rules orientation)
- Engaging   (From self absorbed to concern for others)
- Pleasant   (From irritating to pleasant to be around)
- Straightforward   (From devious to direct and honest)
- Total Score

The BRS is intended to provide a representative picture of the domain of everyday child behavior, and the behavior dimension scores are taken to represent directly observed patterns of strengths and limitations (competency levels) within this domain. The BRS was developed and refined through a process of conducting a number of highly structured small group meetings with people who share children's daily lives (parents, teachers and child care staff), in all numbering about 450. Participants were asked to write down all the observable child behaviors they could think of and then to proceed to delete all item redundancies, trivialities and ambiguities by a process of group consensus. The remaining list was used in 3 separate field studies by approximately 300 adults who completed a total of 1,975 child observations, which were submitted to a series of factor analyses and reliability tests. In brief, the factor analyses produced and replicated the factor structure (item clusters) labeled above as behavior dimensions. Items that did not consistently load at .35 or above on the same factor and below that level on all other factors were deleted. Additionally, items were removed that did not average .75 or above on test-retest interrater reliability studies involving a sample of 40 paired observers and 139 children. Finally, items representing infrequently observed behaviors, that is, behaviors reported to have been observed in fewer than 15 percent of all child observations, across all 3 field studies, were removed as being, by definition, not common to everyday child performance. Interestingly, all of these items were of a problem-oriented type (e.g., was seductive, throws tantrums), and constitute the substance from which CIs, or behavioral "blips" in daily performance, may be operationally defined.

The results of this process suggest that the final version of the BRS form reflects what adults commonly observe in children's everyday behavior and yields reliable reports of observed behavior. Of equal importance, the behavior dimension structure underlying observed behavior has been shown to be stable, and, therefore, a reliable indicator of behavioral patterns. The behavior dimension labels were created by the author on inspection of the item clusters forming each behavior dimension, and submitted to a number of reviewers for their reactions. General agreement was reached on the descriptive adequacy of five labels. The sixth, "Engaging," remains in use, since no consensus could be reached on a superior alternative.

The Task/Social Relations Competency Scale (TSRCS) and Locus of Control Scale (LOC)

The 43 item TSRCS and 26 item LOC scales are child self-report forms. Each is composed of self-descriptive statements of mixed negative and positive phrasing, and associated "True/False" response categories. They are used at entry and release from services, and at any interim point desired, for progressive assessments.

The TSRCS yields a total score and three sub-scores representing competency levels in Task Skills, Peer Social Relations Skills and Adult Social Relation Skills. The LOC yields a single score reflective of sense of self-direction in and responsibility for behavioral performance. The TSRCS was developed by the author, and the LOC was adapted from the Nowicki-Strickland (1973) version of that instrument. Both forms, as presently used, were field tested in a number of studies involving 5,400 and 3,230 children respectively. Each consistently yielded internal consistency reliabilities (Kuder Richardson 20) in the mid-70s or above, correlated modestly with one another (product-moment range: .13 to .30), proved reliable for self scoring by children with third grade reading skills and discriminated between groups, particularly by age at one year intervals or better. (Thomas 1975:65-80, Reichertz 1978:175-207). These results assure reliable child self-report data for use in context with adult observational data.

Score Interpretation

Score interpretation is straightforward. In all cases, higher scores are more favorable than lower scores. In the case of BRS behavior dimension scores, high scores — as contrasted to lower scores — reflect more frequent observance of a greater variety of favorable behaviors, on average, by differing observers from differing contexts. The decision support power of COBRS 2.0 derives from drawing "weight of the evidence" patterns and trends from this multiple observation/viewpoint/time period score matrix which more closely reflects the reality of a child's performance in behavior outcome measurement terms than can be obtained by relying on single measures compared to a single criterion or norm.

2. Types of Reports and Their Application

Reports for behavior dimension score profiles and CI counts may be generated by cross tabulating for categories of up to 10 report variables. To illustrate, a set of 10 report-generating variables is given with user defined variables identified by the (UD) symbol:

- Sex
- Age
- Race (UD)
- Totals
- Living Unit (UD)
- Length of Stay
- School Grade (UD)
- Treatment Classification (UD)
- Prior History (UD)
- Payment Source (UD)

The range of obtainable scores extends from that of a single behavior dimension score for one child to the overall behavior average for an entire client population each quarter.

Weekly Reports. Two forms of weekly tables can be obtained for behavior dimension score profiles for categories of the 10 variables. List tables show the behavior profiles for every child in a category and the averages for the group. Summary tables show only the group averages for all categories of a variable. These options have case assessment and program evaluation applications, respectively. Six- and Twelve-week time trend graphs may also be produced, as needed, to track each and all behavior dimension scores for each child. Finally, Pre/Post and Post/Expected Behavior Analysis Graphs can be produced at case closure, and at interim times, to statistically compare a child's aggregate early (first 12 weeks) to later (subsequent 12 weeks) behavior performance, and to compare performance at case closing (last 12 weeks) to an agency set statistical goal model for determining achievement.

These reports, in conjunction with TSRCS and LOC scores, allow weekly assessments of each child's current performance status by comparisons to both relevant peer group averages and personal time trends and, more broadly, from an overall pre/post gain perspective.

Quarterly Reports. Quarterly tables and time trend graphs for categories of the 10 reporting variables provide behavioral dimension score profiles and CI rates summarized, by week, over 13-week time periods. Quarterly tables also provide separate group average scores for the total caseload, cases opened and cases closed for each category of a variable reported. Finally, a table is produced containing behavior dimension score profiles reflecting the averaged scores reported across all children observed during the entire quarter, for each observer. This table is useful in assessing the orientations toward children of each person who conducts observations.

Taken together, these reports provide information, from a variety of perspectives and at different levels of aggregation, of both immediate and more long range use in case assessment, program evaluation and staff performance monitoring tasks. The capacity of this reporting system to spot trouble before it erupts into harmful, perhaps disastrous, consequences suggests that it is particularly applicable to the critical issue of child maltreatment prevention.

IN CLOSING:
SOME EARLY RETURNS FROM THE FIELD

COBRS 2.0 represents an effort to provide children and youth services with a single, microcomputer supported methodology for meeting a variety of evaluation needs in a reliable, valid, agency adaptive and cost efficient manner. COBRS 2.0 was introduced in early 1987 and was operational, within five months, in practice and test sites in 36 agency locations in 16 different states. Although it is too early to tell how the field will ultimately react to and use the product, we have learned a few things worth sharing during this introductory period from numerous telephone conversations and several site visits with current users.

1. Menu Driven Is Not Enough: Smoothing
the Disjoint Between Program Logic
and Agency Work Rhythms
in the Weekly Data Entry Process

COBRS 2.0 was designed to follow the logic of a weekly data entry routine. Entry dates, grouped for the 52 weeks of the calendar year, are used to consign entered batches of data to their appropriate weekly intervals in the data base. What we have found is that agency work rhythms and the realities of operators' jobs rarely follow this logical sequencing. Sometimes agencies do not collect data every week, and other priorities may result in delays in getting data to the operator. In addition to the destabilizing effects of these lapses, operators must contend with a variety of other complicated duties that may force them to delay data entry, causing two or more weekly batches to pile up, or to assign data entry and report output tasks to a low "catch as catch can" priority.

All of this contributes to the only serious problem yet encountered in implementing the system; namely, operator mismatching of weekly data batches and data entry dates. The most common errors are those of using wrong entry dates for weekly batches entered belatedly and/or a single date when entering several weekly batches at one sitting. In the former case the data are "lost" by consigning them to the wrong week, while in the latter case, whole weekly batches are literally lost by being overwritten while entering succeeding weekly batches. The effect is to impair the sequencing and completeness of the data base and the reports it yields.

To compensate for these distractions, we have adapted the system by incorporating a number of strong reminders on data entry screens and in the Operator's Manual to reinforce the point that, regardless of when weekly data batches are entered or weekly reports are requested, accurate weekly data entry and/or report output dates must be used.

2. COBRS 2.0 Offers Far More Power Than Is Currently Being Put to Use

Briefly put, over the last four years, we listened closely to the recommendations of dozens of informed people including users of the initial 1.2 version and other knowledgeable commentators. In response, we expanded the system's power and flexibility many times over before bringing it to market. The common pattern we find among current users is one of limiting themselves to the more basic aspects of the system. Very little has been tried in the way of adapting the system to specific agency needs. Indeed, very few are even utilizing Critical Incident (CI) counts. A "let's test the water first" guideline is detectable in this, which makes some sense. Getting the basic system up requires little effort and pays immediate dividends, but most of the user options for redesigning system components require higher levels of agency commitment and staff planning. Given these demands and the expertise required to carry out evaluation programs, our experience suggests that there may be merit in offering a basic system and expanding it as user sophistication grows, at least in the field of children and youth social services.

3. How Well Is It Working?
Expected and Imaginative Applications

The basic system is being put to a variety of uses, with some initial success. Conventional applications in various programs include tracking childrens' adaptation in foster family care after release from institutional care; aggregating pre/post findings to support a capital fund raising drive; and, documenting the need for higher state payment rates for certain kinds of behavior problem children. One facility pinpointed a need for improved task skills within a segment of its population and altered its services to meet it. Somewhat more imaginatively, one user has conceived of tracking informal peer groups to confirm or refute their reputations for trouble and another has tested using the BRS to rate staff performance. These are encouraging signs that the range and number of imaginative applications can be expected to expand rapidly as user experience with the system deepens.

REFERENCES

Ainsworth, F. (1985) Direct Care Practitioners: As Promoters of Child Development. *Journal of Child & Youth Care Work 1*(2) 62-70.
Besharov, D. (1985) *The Vulnerable Social Worker.* Silver Springs, MD: NASW.
Combs, J. (1979) An Information System that Measures Foster Casework Effectiveness. *Children Today.* May-June 15-17 & 36.
Fleit, L. (1987) Over Selling Technology: Suppose You Gave a Computer Revolution and Nobody Came? *Chronicle of Higher Education.* April 22, 1987, 90.
Gaylin, W. (1982) The Competence of Children: No Longer All or None. *The Hastings Center Report.* April, 1982, 33-38.

Hambleton, R. (1985) Criterion-Referenced Assessment of Individual Differences. In: C. Reynolds & V. Wilson (eds) *Methodological and Statistical Advances in the Study of Individual Differences*. New York: Plenum 393-424.

Hamburg, D. (1986) Preparing for Life: The Critical Transition of Adolescence. Paper reprinted from *The Carnegie Corporation of New York 1986 Annual Report*. 3-13.

Kent, M. & Rolf, J. (eds) (1979) *Social Competence in Children*. Hanover, NH: University Press of New England.

Krotochwill, T., Mace, F. & Mott, S. (1985) Research Methods for Applied Behavior Analysis. In: C. Reynolds & V. Wilson (eds) *Methodological and Statistical Advances in the Study of Individual Differences*. New York: Plenum 335-392.

Magura, S. & Moses, B. (1986) *Outcome Measures for Child Welfare Services*. Washington DC: Child Welfare League of America.

Maluccio, A. (ed) (1982) *Promoting Competence in Clients*. New York: Free Press.

Mordock, J. (1986) The Inadequacy of Formal Measures of Child Adjustment During Residential Treatment. *Residential Treatment for Children & Youth* 4(2) 55-73.

Mutschler, E. & Hasenfeld, Y. (1986) Integrated Information Systems for Social Work Practice. *Social Work* 31(5) 345-349.

NAFFC Newsletter (1987) Preparing Youth for Independent Living. *1* 1-4.

Nelson, R., Singer, M., & Johnson, L. (1978). The Application of a Residential Treatment Model. *Child Care Quarterly* 7(2) 164-173.

Nowicki, S. & Strickland, B. (1973) A Locus of Control Scale for Children. *Journal of Consulting and Clinical Psychology. 40* 155-158.

Nutter, R., Gripton, J. & Murphy, M.A. Results of a Survey of English Speaking Professional Canadian Social Workers. (1986) *Computer Uses in Social Services* 6(3) 4-6.

Reichertz, D. (1978). *Residential Care: The Impact of Institutional Policies, Structures and Staff on Residential Children*. Montreal, Quebec: School of Social Work, McGill University.

Rimer, E. (1986) Implementing Computer Technology in Human Services Agencies: The Experience in Two California Counties. *New England Journal of Human Services* 6(3) 25-29.

Rindfleisch, N. (1984) *Identification, Management and Prevention of Child Abuse and Neglect in Residential Facilities, Volume 1: Summary and Overview*. Columbus, OH: The Ohio State University Research Foundation. 55ff.

Rubin, E. (1976) The implementation of an Effective Computer System. In: G. Hochman (ed) *Management in Social Welfare: Casebook Studies*. Philadelphia: University of Pennsylvania School of Social Work and the Wharton School. 112-121.

Shyne, A. (1959) *The Use of Judgments as Data in Social Work Research*. New York: NASW

Thomas, G. (1967) *An Assessment of the Evaluation of Effectiveness Guide (EEG).* Madison, WI: Wisconsin Department of Social Services.

Thomas, G. (1975) *A Community Oriented Evaluation of the Effectiveness of Child Caring Institutions.* Athens, GA: RISWR, University of Georgia.

Wilson, D. & Lyman, R. (1983). Computer-Assisted Behavioral Assessment in Residential Treatment. *Residential Group Care & Treatment 1*(4) 25-33.

Hospital Social Work Information System

B. Albert Friedman

KEYWORDS. Hospitals, hospital social work, information systems, health administration, computers, social work practice

SUMMARY. This chapter provides an overview into management information systems used within a hospital social work department. The history of developing the Hospital Social Work Information System (HSWIS) is presented together with a description of the various components of the system. A clear mission statement of the system is also discussed. The use of the system to provide data for a national data base is discussed as well as the present state of the various installations using the system.

GENERAL BACKGROUND

In the hierarchy of a hospital organization, social work departments occupy a unique place. The services these departments provide are not often well understood by many hospital administrators. Hospital administrators, faced with rising health care costs and constrained budgets, must look at every department in the organization and assess the impact each department has on patient care and the cost of providing that care. The services provided by many hospital social work departments are often "invisible." Yet, without the

B. Albert Friedman, EdD, is affiliated with TekniComp Associates, Inc., Dayton, OH; he is a consultant specializing in the design and implementation of computerized information systems for social service organizations. He is also Professor of Computer Information Systems at Sinclair Community College in Dayton, OH. He holds the following degrees: BS degree in Mathematics from the University of Missouri at Kansas City, Masters in Business Administration from the University of Dayton, and a Doctorate in Adult Technical/Vocational Education from the University of Cincinnati.

169

social work department, many vital patient services would be seriously diminished—discharge planning, family and individual counselling, crisis intervention, nursing home placements, etc.

Historically, hospital social work departments have collected very little data about their ongoing operations. However, in the late 1970s and early 1980s escalating health care costs and the federal government's inquiries into the reasons for these escalating costs caused hospital administrators to scrutinize departmental budgets much more closely.

Pressure was exerted on social work directors to provide information about activities in their departments that could be used to determine departmental productivity and costs related to providing services to patients. Social work directors were ill-prepared to supply this kind of information because most social work departments operated autonomously. Social work directors had little or no experience in developing productivity and cost accounting reports or in using these reports as a management tool. They were unused to supplying this kind of information about their departments to administrators.

Because no nationally recognized norms or terminology existed, social work directors could not determine how their departments compared to departments of similar size and activity in other hospitals. Social work directors understood what their workers did but did not know how to convey this information to management. Until pressures for facts and figures mounted, there was no real incentive for social work directors to develop a system to supply the kind of information being demanded by administrators. These pressures formed the impetus to begin quantifying, identifying, and standardizing terminology and to develop a computerized information system—a system vital to the survival of social work departments.

Therefore, in 1975 the Society for Hospital Social Work Directors of the American Hospital Association, decided to develop a model information and measurement system to help their members become professionally accountable.

To achieve this goal, the Society created a task force on accountability whose mission was to identify methods to aid Hospital Social Work Directors in understanding the cost of services and how these costs could be developed. Concurrent with this activity, the

Society also began to investigate the feasibility of developing a standardized reporting system and staffing pattern in hospital social work departments.

In 1983 the Society created another task force to develop a set of concepts and definitions for classifying social work practice. For the first time, information systems currently being used by hospital social work directors throughout the United States were closely examined. The task force's efforts resulted in formulating a set of common data elements, definitions and information modules which were used as part of the computerized management information system developed two years later.

As the work of the task force moved forward, problems were encountered. Most problems involved the way in which social workers conceptualized their workloads. Workloads were carried as open cases or closed cases, or as cases carried forward or reopened. The task force quickly recognized that there was no standardized activity measure. Cases varied from one hospital to another, depending on the size of the hospital, the type of hospital and the skill levels involved in servicing patients. Therefore, the Society appointed a committee to develop a solution based on national inputs. From the inputs received, it was evident that, while most hospital social work directors understood the general concepts about workloads and the skill levels needed to service patients, the directors had no accurate information on the cost of delivering patient services.

Meanwhile, the federal government relaxed its inquiry into health care cost containment. This gave the Society the opportunity to continue their effort toward developing a computerized information system. This effort received top priority by the Society — never again did they want to be caught so unaware.

For this computerized information system to be an effective tool, practice classification was vital. Therefore, the Society appointed a task force whose two main objectives were:

1. Collect examples of information systems being used nationally.
2. Ascertain what kind of information was being collected.

A review of the data collected showed that:

1. A number of hospital social work departments were attempting to gather data to help manage the social work department effectively. Interestingly, the data being collected was fairly consistent throughout the country.
2. Although the data elements being collected was fairly consistent among hospitals, there was lack of agreement among hospital social work departments about how to process the data and use the resulting information to make effective administrative decisions.

Close examination and study indicated a consensus about the basic types of information needed by everyone. Although different departments used different names for the same type of services being delivered and the types of patient problems being addressed, the task force found enough conformity to allow them to classify both services and problems into similar broad categories.

When the task force presented its report to the Society Board in 1983, it was considered an excellent start toward creating a unified approach to solving the information systems problem. The Board published and distributed this report to its members. While it recognized this report was an excellent first start, the Board also recognized that the problem was still not solved. Each hospital social work department would have to decide on a method for collecting and analyzing data — and decide on a method for producing reports from the data collected. The Society recognized that collecting, analyzing and producing reports would place additional workload burdens on social work departments. In addition, the Society was also concerned about the loss of uniformity if each department implemented its own system. Therefore, the Society decided to use the task force report as a starting point to design a computerized information system for use by hospital social work departments throughout the country.

The Society tried an in-house approach to develop a computerized information system, but, since no one had the expertise needed to accomplish the task, the Society contacted an outside consultant for help.

A contract for the design study was awarded to TekniComp Associates, Inc., of Dayton, Ohio, by the Society Board in 1984. Dr. Claudia Coulton of Case Western Reserve was appointed as technical liaison for the project and she worked closely with TekniComp on developing a design document.

A document entitled "A Design for an Automated Hospital Social Work Information System," was published in the fall of 1985. This document became an official publication of the Society for Hospital Social Work Directors and was widely distributed to its membership. Based on the enthusiastic reception of the design document, TekniComp created an operational computer-based information system called the Hospital Social Work Information System (HSWIS). This effort was funded by TekniComp with the cooperation of the Society.

Gaining a better understanding of the Hospital Social Work Information System (HSWIS) requires:

1. Looking at an overview of the system
2. Being aware of the knowledge base required to successfully operate the system
3. Understanding the mission of the system
4. Knowing what the objectives of the system are
5. Examining the operational concept of the system and its components

SYSTEM OVERVIEW

The Hospital Social Work Information System (HSWIS) is designed to assist the hospital social work department in solving their most pressing problems:

1. Managing and controlling daily operations
2. Planning resource utilization
3. Tracking resource utilization
4. Forecasting the demand for hospital social work services
5. Monitoring the impact made by the hospital social worker on patients served by this department

6. Comparing planned activities and outcomes with actual activities and outcomes
7. Meeting hospital social work accountability requirements.

MISSION OF THE HSWIS

The mission of the HSWIS is to provide each user with the ability to determine:

> *Who* provided *how much* of *what* service to *whom* at *what* location, with *what* result, and at *what* cost.

By providing users with these facts, the HSIWS produces all reports required by directors and staff to effectively operate the hospital social work department. This system also provides information to enable hospital administrators and others interested in the work of the department to clearly describe the activities of the hospital social work department and prove its effectiveness in promoting hospital goals.

In addition, the system produces information on floppy disks which are processed at a centralized data center. Reports produced at the data center are used as national norms for hospital social work directors to compare their performance in selected areas against the same indicators in other hospitals.

OBJECTIVES OF THE HSWIS

The primary objectives of the HSWIS are:

1. Maximize the use of limited resources
2. Identify the types and quantities of hospital social work services delivered to specified groups of patients
3. Track patterns of hospital social work services and costs
4. Quantify costs and results of the hospital social work function
5. Develop analytical reports on the intensity and range of hospital social work coverage
6. Track hospital social work department productivity

7. Track and identify patient discharges to see that they are done on a timely basis
8. Improve the quality of care received by patients
9. Collect data on outcomes for targeted problems or patients
10. Determine if all patients in need are being reached by hospital social workers
11. Ensure that priority is being given to high-risk patients
12. Detect social factors that may contribute to excessive costs within the hospital social work department
13. Help resolve social problems
14. Facilitate special statistical studies

OPERATIONAL CHARACTERISTICS OF THE HSWIS

Every hospital department social worker fills out activity reports on each service performed during the work day. Each activity report consists of the following:

1. Social worker identification
2. Patient identification
3. Type of service performed
4. Location where service was performed
5. Time (in minutes) required to perform service
6. Community resource contacted (if applicable)

The system contains both demographic and case data about patients being given care by the hospital social work department, and "ties" this service data to the patient record so that a complete history of all patient activities is maintained by the system. In addition to demographic and service data, the system also contains data about the community resources used by the hospital social work department, the types of services provided by the department, types of patient problems, and types of problem resolutions.

To handle the processing, a keyboard connected to the computer is used for data entry; a printer connected to the computer is used to produce reports; and, a video screen connected to the computer is used to view inquiry results. The system requires a minimal internal memory of 640,000 bytes together with secondary disc storage of 20-30,000,000 bytes for both programs and data.

The system is designed to operate on a variety of computer equipment. It can operate on a desk-top computer as a single-user, single-tasking system, or on a minicomputer in a multi-user, multi-tasking mode. In either configuration, the system can communicate with a mainframe computer and files can be exchanged between the two systems. In addition, the system can be installed on a mainframe computer.

The HSWIS is an on-line system. Therefore, data input to the system immediately updates all files and the system has a current representation of what is happening within the hospital social work department. The reports produced by the system are always up to date and reflect everything that happened within the department since the last time data was input.

The system can produce two types of reports: (1) standardized, pre-defined reports that are delivered with the system, and (2) "ad-hoc" or user-defined reports which are produced by using a report generator integrated into the system. Standardized reports are reports defined by the HSWIS user community as being most useful to every organization. "Ad-hoc" reports are reports required by a specific organization to answer a specific need.

Some of the standard reports produced by the system are:

- Daily Caseload Distribution by Social Worker
- Social Worker Activity by Date
- Productivity Analysis by Social Worker
- Service Cost Analysis by Patient
- Timeliness of Intervention by Social Worker
- Time Standards by Direct Service
- Community Resource Utilization
- Problem Resolution by Social Worker

USER KNOWLEDGE BASE FOR OPERATION OF THE HSWIS

The system, designed for use by those with little or no knowledge of computers, is delivered with documentation so clearly written that people who have never used a computer can install the system quickly and operate the system easily. The documentation includes an overview of computer hardware and software so the user starts at a very primitive level and is brought up to operational status gradually so that both installation and operation are accomplished without any outside assistance. The documentation uses illustrations extensively so that even simple operations like turning on the computer and inserting discs into the disc drives are explained and illustrated.

Using the documentation provided, the system has been sucessfully installed and operated by a large number of people throughout the United States without any assistance or technical support from either TekniComp or the hospital's in-house data processing department.

To effectively use the system, however, hospital social work department directors must have an in-depth understanding of the key indicators which, when integrated into a report, identify both the trouble spots in a department and also the areas where the department's performance is outstanding.

Many managers in social service organizations have difficulty in grasping the power of this type of system. They are not accustomed to using an information system that produces quantitative reports about the activities within their organization. This seems to be true because many management tasks are monitored by instinct rather than by reports. Therefore, systems which are in common use in the "for profit" business sector often cause consternation and upheaval for managers and staff of "non-profit" sector organizations.

Many staff people feel that systems which make them account for their time are going to be used in a punitive way — they are "sure" no system can account for the type of services they provide. Managers in social service organizations seldom have training in the use of quantitative measures and are unsure how to use reports to increase their departmental effectiveness.

Managers of social service organizations will have to increase both their knowledge about computer systems and their professional competence so they can effectively employ advanced management tools like the HSWIS. Knowledge about computers will enable these managers to make the most advantageous use of the system's capabilities — especially in developing "ad hoc" reports. With added professional competence, the manager of a social service organization can utilize the reports produced by the system to increase the effectiveness of the organization by maximizing resources without jeopardizing the quality of patient care.

COMPONENTS OF THE HSWIS

The HSWIS consists of 12 subsystems. Seven are operational subsystems, while the other five are utility subsystems.

The operational subsystems of the HSWIS are:

1. Patient Information Subsystem
2. Service Recording Subsystem
3. Quality Assurance Subsystem
4. Financial Management Subsystem
5. Staff Information Management Subsystem
6. Community Resources Subsystem
7. Social High-Risk Information Subsystem

The utility subsystems of the HSWIS are:

1. Report Generator
2. Financial Modeling
3. Word Processing
4. Statistical Analysis
5. Graphics

All of the operational HSWIS subsystems listed above are used by every installation and permit the system to be "standard" wherever it is used. Since each organization has specific and sometimes unique requirements for identifying its own internal operational codes, the system has 25 tables which can be customized by the individual user. The system can, therefore, be supported on a national basis because all the programs are exactly alike. However, from the user standpoint, the system is customized for appropriateness within a specific installation.

HSWIS INSTALLATIONS

The Hospital Social Work Information System (HSWIS) was installed on a test basis at Akron City Hospital, Akron, Ohio, in July, 1986. In September, 1986, the system was installed and tested in six other hospitals: Massachusetts General Hospital, Boston, Massachusetts; Sinai Medical Center, Detroit, Michigan; Grant Hospital, Chicago, Illinois; St. Lukes Hospital, Kansas City, Missouri; Heartland Hospital East, St. Joseph, Missouri; and Harborview Medical Center, Seattle, Washington.

In addition, the information systems department of the American Hospital Association tested the system extensively to ensure that it operated "bugfree." As a result of this careful testing program, a sophisticated system could be mailed to a large number of inexperienced people and made operational immediately after receipt.

The HSWIS was released nationally in November, 1986. Based on the installation rate during 1987 and 1988, it is anticipated that the total number of installations will reach 400-500 systems.

THE IMPACT OF THE HSWIS ON THE HOSPITAL SOCIAL WORK PROFESSION

As a result of developing the HSWIS, the Society for Hospital Social Work Directors has also developed a list of standard service and problem codes and accompanying definitions which will allow hospital social work directors to compare activities in a variety of different operational areas. Now data from all hospital social work departments can be collected and used to establish a national data base which will, according to professionals in the field, improve hospital social work practice. In addition, as field practice changes, the HSWIS will change to reflect latest developments.

CONCLUSION

In response to the needs of hospital social work departments nationally to become more professionally accountable, to be able to accurately assess the cost of providing services, and to satisfy management's requests for cost accounting information, the Society for

Hospital Social Work Directors of the American Hospital Association appointed several task forces to study problems and provide recommendations. The results of these studies and recommendations culminated in a design document for a computerized information system. With funding on an entrepreneurial basis, TekniComp Associates, Inc. of Dayton, Ohio developed a computerized information system called the Hospital Social Work Information System (HSWIS).

The HSWIS is now successfully installed in a number of hospitals throughout the United States and, within a few years, is expected to be operational in several hundred locations. With the endorsement of the AHA, the HSWIS is expected to become the standard by which systems of this type are judged.

Because the system was designed by members of a national society, it reflects the ideas of the user community, not those of computer professionals. Inherent in the design philosophy of the system is that it always reflect current field practice. Enhancements to the system will be dictated by the user community.

In addition to the implementation of a practical, computerized management information system, the Society for Hospital Social Work Directors of the American Hospital Association has also developed a list of standardized service and problems codes and associated definitions. This outgrowth of system development will allow Society members to gather comparable data on a national basis and establish a national norms data base.

The result of many years of effort by many people has resulted in a system that meets all the objectives of the initial project — a tool to allow hospital social work departments to both survive and grow.

REFERENCE

Friedman, B. A. (1986). *A Design for an Automated Hospital Social Work Information System*. Chicago: Society for Hospital Social Work Directors of the American Hospital Association.

The Personal Computer
and the Small Social Agency

Merlin A. Taber
Louis V. DiBello

KEYWORDS. Computers, social service information system, information management, database

SUMMARY. Use of computers in everyday professional tasks by caseworkers is described. Eighteen front line workers, after two or three hours of training, created and manipulated data bases of client, service, and outcome data tailored to their own caseloads. The authors believe that adoption of computers for everyday tasks by front line workers depends on three elements: Specially designed software which is very user-friendly; conceptual framework as bridge between agency task and computer system; and agency look and feel to all screen displays, forms, and reporting formats. Workers did overcome fear of computers and did see how computers could be professionally useful. This approach seems worthy of examination and further development.

Merlin A. Taber holds a PhD in sociology and is Professor of Social Work in the School of Social Work, University of Illinois at Urbana-Champaign.

Louis V. DiBello holds a PhD in mathematics, directs the Automated Systems Research Group, and is Senior Specialist in Automated Education at the Computer-based Education Research Laboratory on the same campus.

Correspondence may be sent to both authors at 1207 West Oregon, Urbana, IL 61801.

The authors gratefully acknowledge support from Project EXCEL and the School of Social Work of the University of Illinois at Urbana-Champaign; the expert services of Greg Janusz (senior programmer), Dan Weber, Fred Kerr, and and Dan Kao; and especially the good spirits and cooperation of the agency staff who worked with us on this project. Thanks also go to Kathy Proch for editorial assistance.

Computers, that is main frames with their attendant data processing bureaus, have long been a fixture of state human service agencies (Dery, 1981; Carter, 1986). The personal computer has been eagerly taken up by independent clinicians especially for record keeping and test administration (Johnson, 1984; Lynch, 1985; McCullough, Farrell, and Longabaugh, 1986; Meldman, Harris, Pellicore, and Johnson, 1977). Community based non-profit agencies are adopting computers for fiscal records and payrolls and occasionally case data or case decisions (Butterfield, 1986; LaMendola, 1986; Schoech, 1982; Schwab, 1986). However, the personal computer still does not appear on the desk of the front line social worker, nor the small agency program director.

Therefore, with the help of a university grant, a project was designed to encourage front line workers to use personal computers in their daily practice. This article describes the project and its outcomes, identifying what we believe are the necessary prerequisites for workers to use computers for human service tasks.

A DEMONSTRATION PROJECT

The approach tested was to acquaint workers with some new and interesting methods of managing information, in a way that would show immediate gains for them. Three considerations dictated this approach. One, experience indicated that in human services, workers can undermine — or expedite — any administrative information system. Two, human service workers live close to the edge in terms of workload and will not use a procedure that seems intrusive or diverts their energy. Three, and more positively, constant feedback by workers would ensure a more functional system.

The project approach and the project software were tested with 18 direct service workers from twelve community-based agencies with budgets of $200,000 to $2,000,000. These agencies deliver personal social services in local areas and have unreliable funding from a variety of public and private sources. They face the most difficult human problems. The failure of personal computers to penetrate this market, even at giveaway prices, is easy to understand. It should be noted that the workers, while interested in better practice, did not all begin with a desire to learn about computers. They represented a wide range of familiarity and attitude and experience with computers.

The project began by the use of computers for reporting on targeting and productivity to funders. This choice was made for three reasons. First, record keeping and reporting are a heavy burden for small multiply-funded agencies. Any help will translate directly into more worker time for service and improved agency accountability, as well as improved accountability to funders. A second advantage was the advanced state of the database art. Relational database packages are available for use on low cost hardware. The third rationale was the availability of a set of ideas about systematizing client and service recordkeeping facilities (Taber, in press).

Small agency budgets and high workloads require that training, installation, and maintenance costs be very low. Therefore the project team chose to create some new software and procedures for managing case information. The procedures were as close as possible to those already in use, and the software could be run on a small personal computer. The result was a quick-start database for line staff in small social agencies. It was designed so that workers and administrators would see immediate professional products and practical time savings in monthly reporting to funders.

It was planned that the files created for monthly reporting could later be used by staff for caseload and service flow analysis. With hands-on practice, it was thought, agency staff can become critical, non-passive users of technology. The longer term goal was that these professionals become confident in making choices concerning information systems in their agencies.

Previous work has been done on many elements of this kind of approach. The potential, as against actual, uses of computers in social service have been projected by many including Krueger and Ruckdeschel (1985), by LaMendola (1986), by Rapp (1984), by Sircar, Schkade, and Schoech (1983), by Slavin (1982), and by Taber (1975). In social work, the crucial importance of involving end users in planning has also been recognized by many, notably by Schoech (1982, Ch. 10) and by Schoech, Schkade, and Mayers (1981). A case study documenting the need of such involvement is presented by Mutschler and Cnaan (1985). A closely reasoned and highly general argument for attention to professional not computer concerns and to overall integration of information design is presented in Mutschler and Hasenfeld (1986) and Nurius and Mutschler (1984); their conclusions apparently came from work in the university setting but are of wide applicability.

Outside of human services, a low profile, user-guided approach which produced good organizational results, is also described by El Sawy (1985). Attention to work process not just information flow, is also underlined by Drange (1985) for profit organizations. The longer term efficiencies in taking great care to fit systems to organizational culture is well stated by Poertner and Rapp (undated) who call this approach "incremental design."

The authors of this report find strong common themes in these essays and reports: need to integrate office and professional and software routines, absolute necessity of enlisting workers on the front line, and the possibility of small incremental changes toward more rational information management. The authors draw another conclusion from the literature, a conclusion they had independently drawn from their own experience: In system design the hardest part is not writing software but creating an "interface" of ideas, terms, procedures, and software which admits the computer to the work place.

SYSTEM PERFORMANCE CRITERIA

Project guidelines—immediate professional relevance, low start up costs, autonomy of system users—implied several performance standards. Learning time until production of the first professional product had to be low—less than three hours. Training had to feel more like training in practice methods than computer training. For several reasons the software had to be highly user-friendly. Fifteen of the 18 agency staff in the project had no prior knowledge of or even close contact with computers. Wide generality of routines was traded off to gain simplicity for the user. Costly outside consultation, software maintenance services, and outside software developers were not feasible options for these agencies. The system had to permit later editing and additions by agency staff. Otherwise the staff would not experiment with the system on their own.

Software and hardware costs had to be low. Most of the agencies concerned in this project did not have computers. The ones with computers did not own dBASEIII+ or R:BASE or other database packages. The project software should not require agencies to purchase commercial packages. Yet the databases had to be readily transferable, as agency expertise and understanding grew, to any standard package such as dBASEIII+ or R:BASE System V in case the agencies gained access to such software.

SYSTEM ARCHITECTURE

Software and system design as dictated by these performance criteria can be presented briefly under three headings: software design, programming decisions, and hardware selection.

The first decision was that the software have menus and procedures keyed to professional routines. A frame of reference developed by Taber (in press) provided a way to relate databases to practice. This frame of reference supplied terms for an interface that was close enough to agency work routines to be quickly learned. Software functions for workers included setting up and modifying database structures, entering and maintaining data records, and calling for reports as needed. Figure 1 provides a schematic of the software system.

User prompting, on-line help displays, and computer-assisted instruction were programmed to display the same terms and operations found in written instructions and manuals. Database software was designed so that workers could set up three types of databases that were linked together: clients, services, and outcome measurements. These three databases, together with fiscal information were the minimum information needed to adequately describe agency operation. See Figure 2 for a sample agency relational database structure.

Relational databases offer advantages for social services as well as business. The use of linked relational databases simplifies and standardizes data management. In business the capabilities of relational databases have been recognized through the market; relational databases can reduce redundancy in storage of information, simplify procedures for updating records, protect integrity of selected databases, yet permit quick combining of disparate elements (Date, 1986). An application of relational database structures, similar to the one we developed, was prepared for social work practice

FIGURE 1:   SOFTWARE SYSTEM SCHEMATIC

```
DESIGN STRUCTURES
     Create a new Database Structure
     Modify an existing Database Structure
CREATE RECORDS
     Add New Records
     Modify Existing Records
     Delete Existing Records
WRITE REPORTS (Single or Linked Databases)
     Print Database Structure
     Sort and List all Files
     General Breakdown and Summary Reports
          Client Reports
               Single client
                    (including service history and summary)
               Summary Reports
          Service Reports
               Summary by Type of Service
          Outcome Reports
               Summary by Outcome Measurement

UTILITIES AVAILABLE
     Copy, rename, move, delete databases
     Copy database structure only
     Append one database into another
     Import/Export databases to/from other programs
     List (print out) all databases on disk
```

classes at the University of Michigan (Mutschler and Hasenfeld, 1986, and Nurius and Mutschler, 1984).

Following the strategy developed for business, a few linked databases with small numbers of fields in each were planned. Client characteristics, service events, and outcome measurements were set up in three cleanly separated databases linked by one common data element. This separation simplified the underlying computer routines, made it easier for workers to understand the database structures, and allowed for economies in storage as well.

Standardized service and outcome summary reports were explicitly designed into the system. See Figure 3 for an example of a service summary report. These summary reports made it easy to use an accompanying spreadsheet system to compute cost per unit of service.

Ease of use for the worker was more important than generality. For example, the first version of project software provided service and outcome reports for databases of fixed structure, rather than allowing service databases of arbitrary structure and requiring the

FIGURE 2. SAMPLE AGENCY RELATIONAL DATABASE

```
Database 1:  CLIENT
     Fields:
          Client ID (*)
          Name
          Gender
          Age
          Ethnicity
          Presenting Problem
          Legal status of couple relation
          Number of police reports of violence
          Number of children age six or under

Database 2:  SERVICES
     Fields:
          Client ID (*)
          Date of delivery
          Service Type
          Number of Units

Database 3:  OUTCOMES
     Fields:
          Client ID (*)
          Date of observation
          Outcome Type
          Outcome Measure
```

(*) common linking field

FIGURE 3, SAMPLE SERVICE SUMMARY REPORT

SUMMARY REPORT: SERVICES BY TYPE

Agency Name: XXXXXXXXXXX
Databases: CLIENT, SERVICES
Date of Report: September 8, 1987

Service Type =	Ind Couns	Sm Grp	Ref
Number of clients:	23	42	29
Total Number of Units:	335	892	33
Average Units/client:	14.6	21.2	1.1
Range of Units/client:	2 - 35	1 - 62	1-2
Median Units/client:	10	17	1

(*) Abbreviations: Ind Couns = Individual Counseling Session;
     Sm Grp = Small Group Session; Ref = Referral Service.

user to "design" the service reports. This choice — ease of use over generality — was made for two reasons. The first was to promote simple and meaningful databases. The authors believe that most agencies have more data than they use, and that adoption of computers may bury them in unread reports. The second reason was the start-up nature of this demonstration. Agencies and staff learned as they worked. Agency staff could expand or elaborate their databases later as they grew in experience and proficiency.

Two other design considerations were planned for future development but were not attempted during the period being reported here. One was more extensive on-line help and instruction included as an integral part of the package in the form of computer-assisted instruction. The second was a simulation and modeling capability for practice and management decision support. These two are mentioned because they affected the overall programming decisions described next.

PROGRAMMING DECISIONS

The decision was made to program rather than adopt an off-the-shelf software package. Two standard commercial database management packages — dBASEIII+ and R:BASE System V — were considered. Each package had three modes of operation: an interactive mode, a menu-based interactive mode, and a program mode in which the package itself is used to run a program or procedure file.

Problems with Commercial Packages

The interactive mode of either package was rejected as being much too demanding of the user. The interactive mode in each — even with menus — is technical, intricate, and not user-friendly. For example, the menu-based mode in dBASE is called ASSISTANT. ASSISTANT combines pull-down menus and other ideas from LOTUS 1-2-3 and the Macintosh. But the ASSISTANT menus help the user put together the same interactive commands that would have been typed at the dot prompt. A report summarizing amount of service by service type received by various client groups would require the worker to know how to set up or open a database; to issue instructions on indexing of fields in the proper order; to use a query file to establish a filter; and to follow all these steps in the proper order. Workers would not and should not need to maintain the skills required to call up the occasional report using ASSISTANT.

There is a further problem with ASSISTANT. Whenever there are deviations from specified procedures the user is shunted into the general ASSISTANT. Therefore security of agency data would demand that the workers become expert in the ASSISTANT itself, rather than just in a tailored set of reports.

A system with minimal training time, with training that would feel like practice procedures, was needed. It was concluded that adopting dBASEIII + would not work.

What about the menu-based mode of R:BASE called Applications EXPRESS? This mode allows a user to create a menu-based application (equivalent to a procedure file) for a specific set of databases. In other words, without learning how to program in the R:BASE programming language, the worker would end up with a tailored application which would be run through menus. There was another serious problem however. R:BASE Applications EXPRESS, like dBASE ASSISTANT is a fully general and very powerful package. Training time required to master the intricacies of Applications EXPRESS is just as prohibitive — three to five days for someone with computer acquaintance to become a novice, and there would still be no interface to practice. This off-the-shelf package, again, was not satisfactory for our purposes. These analyses demonstrate an important trade-off in system design between ease of use for the worker and power and generality of the system. Greater generality requires the worker to make more complicated decisions and build more intricate constructions.

Choice of Programming Language

The second major programming decision was selection of programming languages. A language was sought which would allow a menu-based and user-friendly database management system to be programmed, and which would not require a great deal of learning time for the programmers.

Both dBASEIII+ and R:BASE System V provide programming languages in which applications can be written. Each language provides built-in database management routines like sorting and scanning; a major programming advantage. A disadvantage however was that any program developed in the project would require the package itself to run the program.

Use of a compiler with one of the commercial packages offered the possibility of combining high user-friendliness with very low cost for installation and maintenance. The compiled program could be written for the small agency environment. The compiled program would be a stand-alone product; the dBASE package would not be required for use of the compiled program. The compiled program files are stored in binary form providing software security.

A dBASEIII+ compiler called CLIPPER was chosen as the primary programming language. This meant that the agencies did not need a commercial database package to run the compiled programs. The compiled programs could be provided to the agencies for the cost of the disks.

Two other languages were used for the code which made database operations accessible to workers. A programming language called TenCORE was used for providing user prompts and a user-friendly shell for the CLIPPER programs. TenCORE was originally developed for producing computer-assisted instruction; it permits highly interactive and user-friendly programs. The "C" programming language was also used for several utility routines, in order to provide "hooks" for later addition of modeling and simulation software.

Hardware Requirements

Hardware requirements for the user were set as low as possible — IBM PC-compatible machines with 256K RAM — no harddisk or math chip required. The software was written to run on these stripped-down personal computers because that was the hardware available to the targeted community agencies. The same considerations ruled out the very user-friendly Macintosh computer. These hardware requirements meant the software ran more slowly and required more disks than would otherwise have been the case; but high user-friendliness was achieved despite these hardware limitations.

FIELD IMPLEMENTATION

The next step was preparation of those parts of the interface other than software. To bring together professional task and computer system, more than a specially designed software structure is required. Professional concepts, screen displays, verbal instructions, forms used to bring in case data, and formats for reports — these also belong to the interface. In addition to software, the interface included written documentation and instruction on organizing and systematizing service record keeping procedures. The final product consisted of 5 program disks and a written set of documentation having many pages of text and 10 planning work sheets.

Workers began actual use of the new procedures and software in four group meetings lasting about five hours each. The workers met in one room and began to use the software for their own purposes. The sessions on computer alternated with individual consultation on database development and use, and feedback from workers on problems they encountered.

The professional task set for the first computer session was to create a computerized client database. Workers created a structure for a client database, printed the structure, and then entered 3 cases and printed out case data. Each worker came prepared with a short list of data items and definitions essential to their program operation. Thus, the first session of about one-half-day exhibited in full the approach of this project. Workers faced the computer — most for the first time — and produced a meaningful professional product before ending the session. They took their disks with them and those that had access to an IBM PC-compatible system could modify, experiment with, or expand their database.

Further steps were carried on in the same fashion. One session was devoted to entering a small client database. Another session was used to create a service database, link the databases and produce reports. One session was spent on fiscal data. In four sessions then the workers had hands-on experience with computers for social service data, learned what databases could produce, and developed rudimentary skills in using a personal computer. At the end of the sessions, the workers returned to their agencies with several disks which contained the three main database structures (client, services, and outcomes) and actual agency data.

PROJECT OUTCOMES

The work reported here is the first phase of a continuing project. It is too early for a formal evaluation. Comment can be made however on progress toward project goals and merits of the approach so far.

The workers generally became more positive toward professional use of computers. A pre- and post-training questionnaire administered to workshop participants showed significant positive gains in attitude. The questionnaire included 48 items each with a 7 category Likert type response, e.g., "Developing computer skills would enhance my social work career." Factor analysis indicated that one factor, with items of heaviest loading having to do with professional uses of computers, accounted for most of the variance. The value of t for increase in mean total score was significant above the .01 level.

Several workers—especially those very enthusiastic at first—became more skeptical. A few hours of experience with actual operation showed them what computers cannot do for their own work, as well as what computers can do. Similar findings—high interest in computers, anxiety about their own performance, skepticism about use of computers for practice—have been reported by Nurius, Richey, and Nicoll (1986) and by Finnegan and Nicoll (1987). In this project the initial computer illiteracy and fear were replaced, for most, by a very positive feeling of at least beginning mastery—the beginnings of functional computer literacy.

Positive change of attitudes, however, was not the main goal of this project. The goal was to initiate use of computers for case information management for working in community based agencies. What then are the prospects for such use?

Written reactions by workers were generally positive toward future use. Several noted that they were asking their agencies to purchase computers. At the other extreme about one-fourth of the workers declared they had learned computers were not for them. Follow-up interviews, however, show some important effects from the half-dozen most enthusiastic of the workers.

Three agencies in which these workers were employed adopted the database package for daily use: a domestic violence shelter, a youth service bureau, and a comprehensive mental health center. Line staff and administrative staff used the database management system for recording and reporting agency program data to funders. These agencies purchased hardware and had small necessary changes made in record keeping procedures.

Was the main goal, to start a process within these agencies toward computerization of professional tasks, achieved? According to the workers, the most powerful motive in adoption, was to meet reporting requirements of funders. However, individual practice, more than agency reporting, was the target in the project. To date, it seems, the use of computers to examine caseload or practice improvement, or to deliver service, has not been realized. It is possible that the use of computers for reporting in these agencies will be institutionalized as part of accountability to funders, without changing work patterns of front line workers.

As to whether a process of agency-directed adoption of new information technology was started, one can only say it is too early to tell. The authors do believe that this professionally oriented approach, with quick-start software, has proven worthy of further attention and development.

DISCUSSION

Following the lead of others, this project sought to make computers a professional tool for information management in the social agency. The project was unusual in its combination of certain elements: Target organizations were small low budget community agencies; approach was through front line workers; a "starter set" of software was programmed to be very user-friendly, yet do professional tasks; close attention was given to all aspects of the interface; and the goal was to make agency staff capable of making choices regarding information systems. In this section, two conclusions, drawn from the work and relevant for human service information management in general, are noted.

The first conclusion concerns knowledge required of end users. The front line social worker is the end user of interest. For these front line workers, computer literacy should consist of using a computer every day for professionally relevant tasks, without knowing anything about how computers work. These interrelated propositions represent a concept extrapolated from the project and worthy of further testing.

The project began with the notion that front line workers can sabotage any administrative system; so why not work directly with them rather than just including one or two on a "user committee?" Once started down that road, it became clear that it was not realistic to expect these workers to learn about computers in general, to practice with DOS commands, or watch demonstrations on what computers could do for them. Human service workers are too overworked and have too many ways to dismiss agency requirements, to engage them in learning without immediate payoff.

So, our first conclusion was that functional computer literacy for agency line workers would be knowing how to turn on the computer and follow instructions on the screen, with those instructions written in familiar language. If one looks at business offices or at accountants' offices where personal computers have had great acceptance, one sees that the system developer has gone to the worker not vice versa. In that sense this conclusion is not at all a new idea, yet it does seem worth mentioning since it has not been clearly articulated for human services.

A second conclusion is that the social service members of the team, not the computer science and programming members, must be in charge. Even technical matters like choice of programming languages and design of system routines need to be cleared for fit to professional procedures and suitability to the work environment. It is not necessary for the social service team members to become programmers. A level of judgement and discrimination are needed and most of all a clear sense of what computers can and can not do. The social service team members must be able to translate operations from the office and the field into administrative procedures, software and sometimes even computer operations.

An example from this project was treading the constant tightrope between more generality and greater ease for the worker. On their own, programmers and technical staff tend to maximize program generality and power at the expense of ease of use. Only a social administrator or experienced practitioner should make decisions about what will work in their agency.

In summary, this project encourages further trials of a start-up, professionally oriented approach. In this project it was possibly to enlist front line workers while keeping a focus on professional not technical questions. Procedures and software were prepared so that workers new to the computer were able to design and enter data-bases after about one-half-day of learning time. Among the agencies employing staff who worked with us, three are continuing to use the software and procedures on their own.

The particular interest of this project, for the authors, lay in the intellectual and organizational as well as technical problems of re-lating information technology to human service technology. Exciting developments are occurring in the personal computer world but the authors are convinced, the big payoffs for human service will come from working on the human service more than the computer end of the bridge.

REFERENCES

Butterfield, W. (1986). Computers changing social work practice. *NASW NEWS*, *31*(10), 3.

Carter, R. (1986). Measuring client outcomes: The experience of the states. *Administration in Social Work*.

Date, C. J. (1986). *Relational Database: Selected Writings*. Reading, MA: Addison-Wesley.

Dery, D. (1981). *Computers in Welfare: The MIS-Match*. Beverly Hills, CA: Sage.

Drange, K. M. (1985, April). Information systems: Does efficiency mean better performance? *Journal of Systems Management*, 22-28.

El Sawy, O. A. (1985). Implementation by cultural diffusion: An approach for managing the introduction of information technologies. *MIS Quarterly*, *11*(2), 131-140.

Finnegan, D. J., & Ivanoff, A. (1987, September). Attitudes toward computer use in social work practice: Does minimal training make a difference? Paper presented at the Human Service Information Technology Applications Conference, Birmingham, England.

Johnson, J. H. (1984). An overview of computerized testing. In M.D. Schwartz (Ed.), *Using Computer in Clinical Practice*, 131-133. New York: Haworth Press.

Krueger, L. W., & Ruckdeschel, R. (Eds.). (1985). Microcomputers in social service settings: Research applications. *Social Work Research and Abstract*, 1985, *21*(4). *The Journal of Social Work*, *30*(3), 219-224.

LaMendola, W. (1986). Software development in the USA. *Computer Applications in Social Work and Allied Professions*, *3*(1), 2-7.

Lynch, D. D. (1985, March). The Computerization of Information Systems in Community Mental Health Centers. (Doctoral dissertation, Chicago). *Social Work Research and Abstracts*, *21*(3).

McCullough, L., Farrell, A. D., & Longabaugh, R. (1986). The development of a microcomputer-based mental health information system: A potential tool for bridging the scientist-practitioner gap. *American Psychologist*, *41*, 207-214.

Meldman, M. J., Harris, D., Pellicore, R. J., & Johnson, E.L. (1977). A computer-assisted, goal-oriented psychiatric progress note system. *American Journal of Psychiatry*, *134*(1), 38-41.

Mutschler, E., & Cnaan, R. A. (1985). Success and failure of computerized information systems: Two case studies in human service agencies. *Adminstration in Social Work*, *9*(1), 67-79.

Mutschler, E., & Hasenfeld, Y. (1986). Integrated information systems for social work practice. *Social Work*, *31*(5), 345-349.

Nurius, P. S., & Mutschler, E. (1984). The use of computer-assisted information processing in social work practice. *Journal of Education for Social Work*, *20*(1), 83-94.

Nurius, P. S., Richey, C. A., & Nicoll, A. E. (1986). Graduate students' experience with, attitudes about, and training interest in computer usage in social work. Paper presented at the Council on Social Work Education Annual Program Meeting, Miami, Florida.

Poertner, J., & Rapp, C. A. (Not dated). Designing social work management information systems. Unpublished manuscript. University of Kansas.

Rapp, C. A. (1984). Information, performance, and the human service manager of the 1980's: Beyond "housekeeping". *Administration in Social Work*, *8*(2), 69-80.

Schoech, D.J. (1982). *Computer Use in Human Services: A Guide to Information Management*. New York: Human Services Press.

Schoech, D. J., Schkade, L. L., & Mayers, R. S. (1981). Strategies for information system development. *Administration in Social Work*, *5*, 11-26.

Schwab, A. J., Jr., Bruce, M. E., & Mcroy, R. G. (1986). Using computer technology in child placement decisions. *Social Casework: The Journal of Contemporary Social Work*, *67*(6), 359-368.

Sircar, S., Schkade, L. L., & Schoech, D. (1983). The database management system alternative for computing in the human services. *Administration in Social Work*, *7*(1), 51-62.

Slavin, Simon (Ed.). (1982). Applying computers in social service and mental health agencies: A guide to selecting equipment, procedures and strategies. [Special Issue]. *Administration in Social Work*, *5*(3/4).

Taber, M. A. (in press). Program design. *Administration in Social Work*.

Taber, M. A. (1975). Information systems for state child welfare agencies: Their promise and their problems. In M. A. Taber, S. Anderson, & C. A. Rapp (Eds.), *Child Welfare Information System* 1-12. Urbana, IL: University of Illinois.

Turem, J. S. (1986). Social work administration and modern management techniques. *Administration in Social Work*, *10*(3), 15-24.

The Continuum of Care System: A Decision Support System in Human Services

A. James Schwab, Jr.
Michael E. Bruce
Susan S. Wilson

KEYWORDS. Decision support systems, computer simulation, child welfare, child placement, decision making

SUMMARY. The Continuum of Care System is a Decision Support System designed to assist social workers responsible for identifying and selecting alternative living arrangements for children unable to remain in their own families. The Continuum of Care System consists of two software packages called MATCH and PROFILE. MATCH produces a rank-ordered list of prospective placement alternatives by statistically comparing an individual child to groups of children previously admitted into different residential facilities. PROFILE summarizes the characteristics and problems of children at each facility in the system.

INTRODUCTION

The Continuum of Care System[1] is a Decision Support System (DSS) designed to assist social workers responsible for identifying and selecting alternative living arrangements for children unable to remain in their own families. The impetus for the Continuum of

A. James Schwab, Jr. is Associate Professor in the School of Social Work, University of Texas at Austin, Austin, TX 78712. He is the consultant for research and software development to the Continuum of Care System.

Michael E. Bruce is the program specialist coordinating the Continuum of Care System for the Texas Department of Human Services.

Susan S. Wilson supervised and implemented data collection for the Continuum of Care System for the Texas Department of Human Services.

199

Care System came from child-placement professionals frustrated by the difficulty in locating appropriate residential alternatives for all children needing out of home care and child-care professionals expected to provide suitable care for children with diverse characteristics and problems.

The Continuum of Care System began as a research project to differentiate children placed in different types of out of home care. This research provided the basis for a DSS to help practitioners sort through the many placement alternatives and, on a case-by-case basis, identify appropriate options for each child. Moreover, the Continuum of Care System gives those who provide residential care a better understanding of the nature of and the number of children needing their services.

The Continuum of Care System evolved as a DSS through the development of two software packages called MATCH and PROFILE. MATCH produces a rank-ordered list of prospective placements by statistically comparing the characteristics of an individual child with the characteristics of groups of children previously admitted into different residential facilities. PROFILE statistically summarizes the characteristics of children in each facility included in the system, indicating where children with specific characteristics and problems have been placed in the past.

THE CONTINUUM OF CARE SYSTEM AS A DSS

The Continuum of Care System falls within the category of computer applications known as Decision Support Systems (DSS). The Continuum of Care System was not developed within the framework of a DSS application; the project had been underway several years before the developers were aware of the term. Nonetheless, the theory of Decision Support Systems provides a good framework for understanding the development and application of the Continuum of Care System.

DSSS have been characterized as *"interactive* computer-based systems that *help* decision makers utilize *data* and *models* to solve *unstructured* problems" (Sprague, Jr. and Carlson 1978). The Continuum of Care System fits this definition. It draws on a data set composed of 133 descriptors for 3460 children in 72 different placements. Both MATCH and PROFILE incorporate models derived from statistics. The MATCH classification model utilizes the statistical technique of discriminant analysis, while PROFILE provides comparisons of means and proportions.

The unstructured nature of child placement decision making has been repeatedly chronicled in the literature (Schwab, Jr., Bruce and McRoy 1984). This unstructuredness has been verified by analyses of the Continuum of Care database which show that most facilities serve children with a wide variety of characteristics. To understand the differences among the groups of children served in various facilities, combinations of characteristics must be examined. There is no simple one-to-one correspondence between individual descriptors of a child and the type of program providing services. Aside from a few behaviors or characteristics involving severe violent acts or disability, there are very few descriptors of a child which by themselves dictate placement only in one specific facility, or even one specific type of facility.

The software package MATCH helps practitioners decide which programs to apply to for residential placement of a child. Based on the characteristics of the child needing care, MATCH provides a list of programs likely to admit the child. MATCH, itself, does not make placement decisions; it simply informs and supports a decision maker.

By identifying those residential programs likely to admit a child, MATCH can reduce the number of inappropriate and unnecessary referrals that might otherwise be made. MATCH may also increase the options available to a child when it lists programs to which a referral might not have been made because the placement worker did not know the program existed.

In addition to providing a definitional framework, the DSS literature identifies five roles that must be filled to develop a DSS: the user who is faced with the decision problem; the intermediary who helps the user, perhaps in entering the data in the computer or acts as a staff assistant; the DSS builder who must have some familiarity with the problem and with information system technology; the technical supporter who adds new capabilities to the system; and the toolsmith who develops the DSS tools and writes the programs for the system (Sprague, Jr. and Carlson, ibid. : 13).

Several of these roles can be vested in one person. For the Continuum of Care System, the DSS builder, technical supporter and toolsmith was one individual. As well, this person had been an administrator of a children's institution and was proficient in information systems technology and programming. In addition, the Continuum of Care staff persons responsible for data collection also functioned in the intermediary role. They trained users to access the system directly and provided access for users with a child to place, but no means of connecting to the computer system.

The list of roles generally cited in the literature does not include an activity viewed as critical to the implementation of a DSS like the Continuum of Care System. The introduction of a new system of information processing, whatever its scope, is a form of organizational and inter-organizational change. The problem to be solved may not be new to the organization, but the DSS may supplant previous solution methods. Such a change contains a political component requiring management skills associated with coordination of diverse organizational and interorganizational actors who are needed to provide and share information.

Also critical to the acceptance and use of a DSS is the user-interface which involves a dialog between the user and the DSS. "Even if a DSS provides extremely powerful functions, it may not be used if the dialog is unacceptable" (ibid. : 198). The alternative dialog forms include question-answer dialogs, command language dialogs, menu dialogs, input form/output form dialogs, and various combinations. Deciding which form of dialog to use involves trade-offs between the requirements placed on the user of the system and the requirements placed on the system designer and programmer. The easier a system is to use, the harder it is to design and program. The design/use decisions made in the development and implementation of the Continuum of Care System are discussed in greater detail below.

A BRIEF HISTORY

The Continuum of Care System began as a pilot research project to study the relationship between the characteristics of children needing out of home care and the alternative facilities providing out of home care such as foster families, group homes, basic child care programs, and residential treatment centers. By understanding this relationship, we could attempt to model decisions to place children into different residential programs based on known client characteristics.

Like the intake or diagnostic process in any type of human services, the child placement process requires an assessment of client characteristics and service alternatives. This assessment is necessary to insure that the child for whom placement is being sought is referred to a service alternative appropriate to his or her needs.

The placement process can be viewed as a classification problem in which client characteristics are related to one of the available service alternatives. Typically the placement decision is made in terms of categories of residential child care programs established by licensing agencies, such as foster family care, basic child care, residential treatment, etc.

The difficulty in selecting the most appropriate type of residential care for a particular child can vary substantially. For example, a young child needing temporary residential care while a parent recuperates from an illness will clearly need a very different type of residential program than a juvenile offender who requires long term care in a highly structured setting. However, the selection of the appropriate residential program for the juvenile offender becomes less obvious when the choice for placement requires selecting between a private community treatment center, a group home for delinquents, or a state reform school.

Prior to the Continuum of Care System, another research project (Jaffe 1979) on child placement decision making developed a computer model that cumulated the recommendations of placement workers about where a child with specific characteristics should be placed. A very weak correspondence between worker recommendations and actual placement decisions led to the conclusion that a model produced in this way did not yield an effective tool for placement planning.

Instead of asking placement experts to articulate their criteria for child placement decisions, the Continuum of Care System approached the problem by focusing on children for whom placement decisions had already been made. This approach involves an inductive analysis that attempts to reproduce actual, known decisions for as many cases as possible.

The analysis utilized a database of client characteristics extracted from the written intake materials for a sample of 50 children and adolescents recently admitted to each of the facilities included in the pilot study. The intake materials were assumed to represent the assessment information available to decision makers at the admitting residential programs at the time the decision was made to accept the child into the program. The database consisted of 133 items which measured the demographic, familial, emotional, behavioral, educational, and prior treatment characteristics of children who were grouped together on the basis of having been admitted to a particular facility.

The statistical technique used to associate known placement decisions and client characteristics was discriminant analysis, a multivariate technique which produces a set of mathematical functions that maximizes the difference between the known groups of subjects, or children placed in each program.

The mathematical functions produced by the discriminant analysis were used to predict which program each of the subjects had been admitted to. The correspondence between actual admission and predicted placement provides a measure of the accuracy or usefulness of the statistical model for child placement decision making. An accurate discriminant model can be used as a basis for predicting or recommending placement alternatives for children not included in the original sample.

The accuracy rate for the discriminant model using the seven institutions in the pilot study was 69%, an acceptable rate for models with this number of alternatives (Schwab, Jr., Bruce and McRoy 1984). Based on this result, the Continuum of Care Study was funded as an ongoing research project to expand the number of facilities included in the study and to develop computer software that converted the statistical model into decision support tools for practitioners involved in child placement.

In the five-year period since the study went from being a pilot study to an ongoing research project, the model has grown to include assessment information on samples of children and adolescents admitted to 72 residential programs. Included in the 72 samples are children who were placed with adoptive families, foster families, group homes, basic child care facilities, residential treatment centers, state hospital programs for children and adolescents, and state reform schools for delinquents. Measuring the accuracy of the model's placement recommendations for such a large number of samples is a complex problem. Difficulties arise because the definition of an accurate, appropriate placement recommendation may include more than a single program (Schwab, Jr., Bruce and McRoy 1985).

Most of the placement recommendations generated by the model were comparable to those made by locally acknowledged experts in child placement. In situations where a lack of agreement was found between the recommendations generated by the model and the recommendations made by placement experts, errors were also found in the child's assessment information input to the model. Following the "garbage in, garbage out" principle, inaccurate assessment information entered into the model resulted in inaccurate placement recommendations. This experience demonstrated that the data entry process to the model should contain multiple checks to detect and enable correcting incomplete or inconsistent client assessment information.

Given statistical and practitioner validation of the accuracy and utility of recommendations produced by the discriminant model, a computer program called MATCH was developed to make this information easily available to practitioners. Before proceeding to a discussion of MATCH, one criticism of the entire approach underlying its development will be addressed.

The modeling approach used in the Continuum of Care Study is subject to a criticism for which no effective response is available. Modeling an existing service system may include ineffective placement decisions as well as effective placement decisions. The model cannot differentiate between the two. Any flaws that exist in the current system of care will be reflected in a model of that system of care.

One solution to this problem is to have all computer generated placement recommendations reviewed by experts sensitive to the possibility that a given recommendation may be inappropriate. If recommendations are made directly available to workers through an interactive computer program, this solution is ineffective since an expert is not likely to be present and some users have only limited knowledge of the child placement system. The net result is that inappropriate recommendations could lead to inappropriate referrals—the very problem that the system attempts to alleviate. Inappropriate referrals should not, however, result in inappropriate placements because the decision to admit a child into a program rests with institutional decision makers and placement practitioners, and not with a model that offers recommendations.

MATCH

The development of the computer software to provide placement recommendations for a child evolved through several stages of software development and revisions until the current format was produced. Recommendations can be made both for children not included in the original database, i.e., not currently in placement at one of the institutions contained in the discriminant model, and for children in the database whose characteristics have changed sufficiently to warrant a new set of recommendations.

The first placement recommendations made by the Continuum of Care System were computed by the *Statistical Package for the Social Sciences* (SPSS) (Nie, et al. 1975) which was used to develop the original discriminant model. Using the SPSS computer package as the vehicle for obtaining placement recommendations had two major drawbacks. First, SPSS could not be used by most practitioners. A computer programmer/statistician was required to obtain placement recommendations from the system. Second, SPSS output provided only the two highest recommendations for a case which it classified. Two recommendations are often insufficient since the recommended institutions may or may not have a vacancy available at the time.

While SPSS was invaluable in the development of the discriminant model and is still used for ad hoc analyses and verification when new models are built, it became obvious that a specific program would have to be developed which was easy to use and which quickly provided a longer list of recommendations.

A computer program[2] for data entry was designed to enable project staff to interactively enter assessment information at a computer terminal. The characteristics or descriptors of the child for whom placement recommendations were being sought were indicated by typing in a series of three letter codes. While this worked sufficiently well for project staff, it exposed one of the most prevalent problems in designing interactive software for professionals in any human service field — the lack of touch typing skills. Placement workers who tested the program found it to be slow and tedious because typing three letter codes to enter information was awkward and error-prone. The net result was that workers, already intimidated by computers, were reinforced in their fears about computers because the program required typing skills that were not consistently available. Eliminating the need to type in three letter codes became a priority for the next version of the software.

The format for the display of recommendations on the computer terminal screen was designed during the development of this version and remains virtually the same despite extensive revisions to other sections of the software. It was decided that the output of MATCH would list the ten top placement recommendations for each child, instead of only the two provided by SPSS. The number ten was selected as a reasonable number of choices to assure that at least one of the recommended placements would have a vacancy.

As shown in the sample output screen in Figure 1 below, the ten placement recommendations generated by the model are ranked in order by the probability scores listed in the column labelled "Forced Ranking Among All Groups." The first column of probability scores, "Similarity to This Group Only," indicates the chances that the child has for admission to each of the 10 residential programs listed in the left-hand column.

Figure 1.

CONTINUUM OF CARE PLACEMENT MATCHING REPORT: 18 MAR 84

MODEL 1: ALL VARIABLES FROM ADMISSION RECORDS/ALL CASES IN ALL BENEFIT GROUPS

INSTITUTION OR PROGRAM RECOMMENDED FOR THIS CHILD	SIMILARITY TO THIS GROUP ONLY	FORCED RANKING AMONG ALL GROUPS
CENTRAL STATE TREATMENT CENTER	.9995	.4060
CENTER FOR GIRLS	.9835	.3312
CHURCH CHILDRENS CENTER	.8418	.1178
TEEN TREATMENT CENTER	.8086	.0606
SOUTHWEST CHILDRENS HOME	.1204	.0250
EASTERN CHILDRENS HOME	.5910	.0140
NORTHWEST CHILDRENS HOME	.3696	.0138
CITY CHILDRENS HOME	.7724	.0118
CHURCH CHILDRENS HOME	.1497	.0050
FOUNDATION TREATMENT CENTER	.0933	.0038

CODES: C=CHANGE ITEM N=NEXT SCREEN P=PRIOR SCREEN Q=QUIT R=REDO LINES

An accurate interpretation of the list of recommendations requires the use of both probability scores. If a child is very similar to the children admitted into several residential programs, then the probability scores in the column labelled "Similarity to This Group Only" will be high and can be used as the basis for placement recommendations. However, if the child has a very unique set of needs and is characterized as being "difficult to place," then the child will have very low probability scores in the "Similarity to This Group Only" column. A low score in the "Similarity to This Group Only" column indicates that the child is not similar to the children admitted to any of the 72 residential programs in the model. Since the child must still be placed somewhere, the probability scores in the column labelled "Forced Ranking Among All Groups" guide the selection of the top recommendations.

Whether or not probability scores should be included in an output display along with the list of recommended programs has been the subject for debate among project staff. Feedback from users indicated that the probability scores should be left in. Many felt that the numbers were helpful in interpreting the results and they were comfortable in using them; those who saw them as confusing tended to ignore them anyway and only look at the list of recommended programs.

The next version of MATCH revised the data entry software from requiring a three letter code to marking an "X" beside all descriptors on the terminal screen which characterized the child for whom placement recommendations were being sought. A few descriptors required a numeric response, e.g., number of prior placements in a foster home, or a date entry, e.g., date of birth. The data entry software printed four successive lists of child assessment descriptors on the terminal screen, and the user was led through all descriptors sequentially by positioning the cursor at the next item. After all data items that described a child were entered, the computer calculated a set of recommendations and displayed the top ten in the format shown in Figure 1.

After a short while, users suggested that it would be helpful if they were able to move freely between screens of items, and between descriptors on different screens. Since users found it difficult to be completely certain that each item entered applied to the child, users requested that the software allow them to return to the data entry screens after viewing recommendations to change an item and have the computer re-calculate the recommendations. Users could then examine the impact of the changed item on the set of recommendations provided.

These revisions were incorporated in the current version of the data entry software, producing data entry screens similar to the one shown below in Figure 2.

The screen has been completed to indicate what it would look like for a hypothetical case of a seventeen-year-old girl in the conservatorship of Child Welfare, who was the second oldest child in a family where the parents are no longer married and their rights terminated.

The bottom line of the display shows the single character codes which can be entered at any time to satisfy the movement requirements requested by users. The codes "N" and "P" enable the user to move between the data entry screens. The code "C" enables users to move between descriptors on the same or on another data entry screen. The code "C" also appears on the recommendation screens as shown in Figure 1 above, enabling users to jump back to the data entry screens to change or correct an item.

Figure 2.

```
 SEX:              I ETHNICITY:          I DATE OF:
   (1) --MALE      I (3) --MINORITY       I (5) BIRTH:  12 MAR 69
   (2) X-FEMALE    I (4) X-NON-MINORITY   I (6) FIRST PLACEMENT:  15 MAR 69
 ---------------------------------------------------------------------------
 CONSERVATOR:          I LEGAL STATUS:             I PARENTS MARITAL STATUS:
   (7) --FAMILY MEMBER I (11) --DEPENDENT/NEGLECTED I (15) --NEVER MARRIED
   (8) X-CHILD WELFARE I (12) --CHINS              I (16) --INTACT MARRIAGE
   (9) --TYC          I (13) --DELINQUENT          I (17) X-MARITAL BRKDOWN
  (10) --JUVENILE DEPT I (14) --COMMITTED [NON-TYC] I
 ---------------------------------------------------------------------------
 FAMILY DESCRIPTORS:                (25) --FAMILY IS POOR
  (18) X-PARENTAL RIGHTS TERMINATED (26) --PARENTAL CRIMINAL ACTIVITY
  (19) --UNSTABLE RELATIONSHIPS     (27) --PARENT ON PAROLE/IN PRISON
  (20) --FATHER MENTALLY ILL OR MR  (28) --FAMILY CONFLICT/VIOLENCE/SEX ABUSE
  (21) --MOTHER MENTALLY ILL OR MR  (29) 1--NUMBER OF OLDER SIBLINGS
  (22) X-FATHER PHYSICALLY ILL      (30) 2--NUMBER OF YOUNGER SIBLINGS
  (23) --MOTHER PHYSICALLY ILL      (31) ---NUMBER OF SIBS PLACED OUT OF HOME
  (24) --PARENT SUBSTANCE ABUSER    (32) ---NBR SIBS TO PLACE WITH THIS CHILD
 ===========================================================================
 DIRECTIONS:  THIS SCREEN IN NOW COMPLETE.  IF YOU WISH TO MAKE ANY CHANGES,
 ==========   ENTER C AND RETURN.  IF THE SCREEN IS CORRECT, HIT RETURN.
 ===========================================================================
 CODES: C=CHANGE ITEM   N=NEXT SCREEN   P=PRIOR SCREEN   Q=QUIT   R=REDO LINES
```

The code "R" rewrites the current data entry screen which can become garbled by noise on the phone lines used to connect the interactive user to the computer. The "Q" option provides the user with a means for exiting the program at any time. The user is given an opportunity to reverse a "Q" command if entered inadvertently.

Directly above the line of codes are two lines for directions explaining what the computer is expecting the user to do next. The direction lines are updated automatically so that they always contain the correct instructions for the descriptor at which the cursor is positioned. This area of the screen is also used for error messages in data entries. The definition of what constitutes an erroneous entry was relaxed to accommodate the needs and habits of individuals where possible. For example, the user is directed to enter dates in the form "2 DEC 86," but the program will accept dates in the forms "12/2/86" or "December 2, 1986," since the user's intention can be interpreted easily. To require a practitioner to re-enter information that can easily be interpreted promotes the view that computers are demanding, unfriendly taskmasters.

While practitioners learn the technical aspects of using MATCH rather quickly, confusion about the meaning of a specific descriptor requires more extensive training and has resulted in a written set of instructions that includes definitions and examples for each descriptor. In a future version of MATCH, this information will be available to users as part of the computer program so that they can access it interactively as needed. Whether the information is available in a manual or on the computer, confusion about the meaning of descriptors will continue until a common set of descriptors and their meanings are adopted by all practitioners.

In addition, more checks should be included for contradictory or missing information, such as an unusual grade level in school for a child of a certain age, e.g., a sixteen-year old in the sixth grade. While the information entered may in fact be correct, an erroneous entry or omission can produce inappropriate recommendations.

MATCH was designed to be used directly by practitioners and in many instances it is. In agency units where workers are not comfortable with computers, they often prefer to mark descriptors on a paper version of the data entry screens, and have a clerk or secretary actually enter the data items on the computer terminal. It is expected that interactive usage by workers will increase as practitioners become more accustomed to working with computers.

PROFILE

While MATCH answered the question of where to seek placement for a specific child with certain characteristics, it did not answer the following related questions: What characterizes the children placed at each of the 72 residential programs in the system? Which programs have taken children with particular characteristics such as fire-setting, running away, aggression, suicide attempts, etc.?

To answer such questions, a second software program named PROFILE was developed. PROFILE analyzes the same data base as MATCH, but in a different way that provides answers to these questions.

The first version of PROFILE was written at the same time as the first release of MATCH. It requires a user to type four-letter abbreviations to request information as shown in Figure 3 below.

This program is generally used only by project staff who were not dismayed by the typing requirements for eliciting output from the program. A user is presented menus like that in Figure 3 to select from.

Figure 3.

```
INDICATE THE  DEMOGRAPHIC/CHILD ABUSE VARIABLES
YOU WANT BY ENTERING THE CODE FOLLOWING THE NAME.

TO INCLUDE    SEX IS MALE            ENTER:    MALE
TO INCLUDE    ETHNIC MINORTY         ENTER:    ETHN
TO INCLUDE    AGE FIRST PLACEMENT    ENTER:    AGE1
TO INCLUDE    AGE AT PRESENT TIME    ENTER:    AGE
TO INCLUDE    TIME SPENT PLACEMENT   ENTER:    TIME
TO INCLUDE    DIAGNOSED PSYCHOTIC    ENTER:    PSYC
TO INCLUDE    DISTURBED NON-PSYCHO   ENTER:    DIST
TO INCLUDE    IQ BELOW SEVENTY       ENTER:    IQLO
TO INCLUDE    NEGLECT                ENTER:    NEGL
TO INCLUDE    EMOTIONAL ABUSE        ENTER:    EMOT
TO INCLUDE    PHYSICAL ABUSE         ENTER:    PHYS
TO INCLUDE    SEXUAL ABUSE           ENTER:    SEXU

         TO INCLUDE ALL OF THE ABOVE      ENTER:    ALL

     AFTER YOU HAVE MADE LAST CHOICE      ENTER:    END
```

PROFILE permits the user to select residential programs and client descriptors in a desired order. It also enables a user to form groups of institutions so that, for example, one specific residential treatment center can be compared to the aggregate group of all other residential treatment centers.

Output from PROFILE consists of the average score for each characteristic selected for each institution selected, as shown in Figure 4. If the characteristic selected is numeric, this score is the arithmetic average. If the characteristic selected is a descriptor, this score represents the proportion of persons who have the characteristic. Output is available interactively at the terminal screen, printed on computer paper, or both.

A new version of PROFILE is underway. The entries required by the user to request information will follow the model employed in MATCH. More importantly, the output will be structured as bar charts to facilitate comparisons of characteristics across institutions or groups, as shown in Figure 5.

With a graphic output display, the user can identify at a glance which programs tend to admit children who have particular characteristics. The information on the graphic chart is the same information contained on the eighth line of the previous display, but in a form that is easier to read.

Other changes and features to PROFILE are planned. The output format may be changed to indicate the number of children in the sample for a program and the date on which the assessment data

Figure 4.

	WESTERN BOYS RANCH	RURAL GROUP HOME	DOWNTOWN SUP APRTMT	EAST GROUP HOMES	EAST RESID INTERVENTN
SEX IS MALE	1.00	1.00	.50	.42	.40
ETHNIC MINORTY	.21	.56	.30	.70	.76
AGE FIRST PLACEMENT	12.19	13.01	11.55	11.01	13.62
AGE AT PRESENT TIME	15.30	14.01	16.69	13.26	15.51
TIME SPENT PLACEMENT	3.11	1.00	5.14	2.25	1.89
DIAGNOSED PSYCHOTIC	0	0	.02	0	0
DISTURBED NON-PSYCHO	.83	.77	.64	.14	.24
IQ BELOW SEVENTY	.02	.14	.04	0	.02
NEGLECT	.79	.84	.72	.66	.78
EMOTIONAL ABUSE	.05	.05	.08	.14	.04
PHYSICAL ABUSE	.36	.19	.32	.16	.30
SEXUAL ABUSE	.02	.05	.16	.08	.08
SEVERE ABUSE/NEGLECT	.17	.14	.24	.22	.20

ENTER B OR BACK, F OR FORWARD, E OR EXIT   <<SCREEN   1 OF   2 >>

Figure 5.

```
                                                          PAGE   7 OF  13
ENTER CODE LETTER OF CHOICE:
     N=NEXT PAGE  P=PRIOR PAGE   G=GO TO PAGE   R=RETURN   H=HELP   Q=QUIT

                              IQ BELOW SEVENTY

WESTERN BOYS RANCH    (  2%)  !=
RURAL GROUP HOME      ( 14%)  !=======
DOWNTOWN SUP APRTMNT  (  4%)  !==
EAST GROUP HOMES      (  0%)  !
EAST RESID INTERVENT  (  2%)  !=
SOUTHWEST CITY HOME   ( 16%)  !========
TEEN SHELTER          (  0%)  !
ONE HALFWAY HOUSE     ( 11%)  !=====
TWO HALFWAY HOUSE     ( 13%)  !======
                              !----+----+----+----+----+----+----+----+----+----+
                              0   10   20   30   40   50   60   70   80   90  100
```

was collected. Finally, characteristics that show statistically significant differences among groups will be marked with a symbol like an asterisk, as an additional aid in comparing institutions. PROFILE will make available, on a routine basis, comparisons that now require ad hoc analyses.

SPECIAL ANALYSES

The programs MATCH and PROFILE were developed for interactive use as information systems that would be used by practitioners. Given the magnitude of the database that was constructed to support these applications, it was anticipated that questions would be posed for analyses which are more related to policy and budget issues, and which are not a routine part of the Continuum of Care System activities. For such requests, SPSS and other standard statistical packages are used to conduct the analysis.

One type of analysis that is fairly common is the statistical comparison of the characteristics of children who are placed in treatment facilities by different state child-placing agencies. Similarly, the comparison between the children that a state agency places in its own treatment centers versus the children the agency places in private treatment centers has been requested on several occasions.

These analyses are frequently motivated by concern with the way child-care budgets are spent or the fairness of reimbursement rates for private programs. While it is usually assumed that higher rates are paid for children with more complex problems, the statistical evidence regarding this contention is ambiguous. Programs accept children with a range of problems, so that an individual child could potentially be included in the range of two different programs whose cost of care are quite different.

Different classification systems based on a single database may be required to meet different needs. Regarding issues of reimbursement rates, the Continuum of Care System has been involved with other public and private organizations in efforts to develop a "level of care" classification system for children in placement programs. The underlying premise for this type of classification model is that the rate of reimbursement should be associated with the level or intensity of services required to respond to a child's individual needs. While the database was not specifically developed to answer such questions, it is currently the only database which includes the characteristics of individual children available for such an analysis.

The final policy question in which the Continuum of Care System has frequently been involved attempts to answer the question of where a group of children could be served if the program in which they are currently placed were no longer available. For this analysis, the database is used as a simulation model of the child-care system in the state. SPSS is used to construct a new discriminant model of the institutions remaining in the system. Based on the discriminant model, the cases in the facility no longer available are classified among the remaining facilities.

This analysis may ultimately be the most important contribution that a system like the Continuum of Care can offer, as a tool in analyzing needs and shaping the resources provided for the care of children in a geographic region.

CONCLUSION

The Continuum of Care DSS was called upon to assist in the placement of approximately 600 children in the past two years. Though it was envisioned as a system that would be directly accessed by practitioners, its more frequent use has been via telephone calls to project staff who enter the child's characteristics into the computer and report back the recommendations.

Anecdotal evidence further indicates the degree to which the Continuum of Care System is supportive of decision making in child placement. From the perspective of facilities participating in the system, PROFILE has been used to document budgetary requests. Statistical evidence can be used to supplement arguments that the children served in a particular facility represent a unique segment of the population needing care.

Numerous cases have been reported in which a successful placement was initiated by a MATCH recommendation to a facility that was previously unknown to the placement worker. In addition, the power to simulate different characteristics for a child was demonstrated by a child welfare supervisor unable to obtain placement for a child in her conservatorship who had been involved in many delinquent acts. This supervisor demonstrated to a juvenile judge how the scarcity of resources she encountered evaporated and additional placement alternatives were available, if the child's conservatorship was changed to the state agency whose resources were devoted to the needs of delinquent youth.

The computer tools developed by the Continuum of Care System have focused on assisting human service practitioners in children's services. These tools are viewed as generically applicable to a variety of services where the desired mix of services or the treatment plan is based upon a diagnostic classification decision, such as placement alternatives for the mentally ill, the mentally retarded, the elderly, or the unemployed. Eventually, the matching process may provide decision support for assigning individual clients to workers so that each client receives help from the worker with the greatest probability of providing effective services for a particular complex of problems.

NOTES

1. The Continuum of Care Project has been funded by the Texas Department of Human Services through state grant funds from the National Center for Child Abuse and Neglect under P.L. 93-247.

2. The computer program was written in the FORTRAN programming language, using a statistical subroutine library developed by International Mathematical and Statistical Libraries, *IMSL Library: Reference Manual* (Houston, Texas: IMSL, Inc., 1979).

REFERENCES

1. Eliezer D. Jaffe, "Computers in Child Placement Planning," *Social Work*, 24 (September 1979), pp. 380-385.

2. Norman H. Nie, C. Hadlai Hull, Jean G. Jenkins, Karin Steinbrenner, and Dale H. Bent, *SPSS: Statistical Package for the Social Sciences* (New York: Mc-Graw-Hill Book Co., 1975).

3. A. James Schwab, Jr., Michael E. Bruce, and Ruth G. McRoy, "Matching Children with Placements," *Children and Youth Services Review*, 6 (Spring 1984), pp. 125-133.

4. A. James Schwab, Jr., Michael E. Bruce, and Ruth G. McRoy, "A Statistical Model of Child Placement Decisions," *Social Work Research and Abstracts*, 21 (Summer 1985), pp. 28-34.

5. Ralph H. Sprague, Jr. and Eric D. Carlson, *Building Effective Decision Support Systems* (Englewood Cliffs, New Jersey: Prentice-Hall, Inc., 1982), page 4. See also: Peter G. W. Keen and Michael S. Scott Morton, *Decision Support Systems: An Organizational Perspective* (Reading, Massachusetts: Addison-Wesley Publishing Company, 1978).

SECTION IV:
ADVANCED APPLICATIONS:
INFLUENCING THE FUTURE
OF HUMAN SERVICES

Introduction

As advances in computer technology and the accompanying software development are made, new perspectives for envisioning changes in human services emerge. Older perspectives focused positively on the computer as if it were simply another labor saving device of the consumer product revolution, while on the negative side, the invasiveness and anti-humanism of computers, and the phenomenon of "garbage in, garbage out" were used to challenge the utility of the new machines and their proper place in the human service environment. Now, the increased accessibility and power of the computer to aid in daily activities and decision making provides a vision of an emerging partnership between computers and human service workers—a partnership where the computer is both ubiquitous and invaluable to the work place, and acts as an extension of our knowledge and thought.

In this section one finds aspects of such a human service perspective given to each of the following: artificial intelligence (especially in the prototypical frameworks of expert systems and decision support systems), Markov processes in operational research, assessment methodology, and causal thinking.

While much of this material may be new to many, the work often shows a debt to other fields, such as business, engineering, medicine, social planning, and military defense, where these concepts have been implemented in well developed applications. The present offerings exemplify the creative and often difficult task of translating concepts developed within other spheres to the purpose of solving persistent problems and of opening new frontiers in human service practice.

Of these examples, Expert and Decision Support Systems (DSS) are especially interesting in their use of human service knowledge. In our own experience, an Expert System (ES) or a DSS actually forces a developer to systematically organize the expert knowledge and reasoning in a manner that can cause a clarity and insight that didn't previously exist. The use of ES shells can also create a more friendly, time saving environment for a developer than the use of a programming language. Although ES shells have some limitations, they have the impact of making the computer a more transparent device, allowing a person to focus more of his or her attention on the human services knowledge and its relation to the problem at hand.

Expert and Decision Support Systems are perhaps the most obvious of computer programs in their use of human services knowledge. However, many other programs — such as data bases — also demand that one clarify and organize the relationships of concepts, goals, and procedures before the computer can become an effective partner. Therefore, computer development should be viewed not only as an opportunity for individuals and organizations to learn more about computers, but also as an opportunity to engage in a human services oriented developmental process.

In this respect, these articles may stimulate readers to continue this exploration of the intersections of computer concepts and their human services application. While the articles presented touch a number of important points in this conceptual continuum, much creative work still needs to be done. It is within this area of creative development that we urge individuals with the highest proficiency in human service to lend their abilities.

Expert Systems: New Tools for Professional Decision-Making

Wallace J. Gingerich

KEYWORDS. Computers, expert systems, artificial intelligence, expertise, decision-making, human services, mental health, problem selection, knowledge acquisition, knowledge representation, tools

SUMMARY. Expert systems are computer programs which embody the expertise of a human expert in order to consult and advise on a specific problem. It is now becoming feasible to apply expert systems technology to problems in the human services. This article describes what expert systems technology is and how it may be applied in human service practice. Finally, some of the promises and pitfalls of this new technology are addressed.

Mr. Vanguard, a brief family therapist (de Shazer et al., 1986; de Shazer, 1985), has just completed the first portion of an initial interview in which a young woman, Mary Jones, reported a history of cocaine abuse, but a strong desire to stop. Ms. Jones is already doing several things to help her stop using cocaine (unplugs her phone, does not go out with her friends, knits and watches TV to keep her mind off her desire to get high), but she is unsure she can

Wallace J. Gingerich, MSW, PhD, is Associate Professor, School of Social Welfare, University of Wisconsin-Milwaukee. His main teaching and research interests are in the areas of clinical practice, clinical evaluation, and computer applications in the human services. Recently he has been involved in developing an expert system to advise family therapists on intervention design. Dr. Gingerich is also a practicing social worker and family therapist.

keep it up. Ms. Jones also reported that she relies on her parents and friends to help her finance her habit.

Before deciding what homework task to give his client, Mr. Vanguard goes next door to consult with BRIEFER, a demonstration prototype expert system (Goodman, 1987). Excerpts of the consultation with BRIEFER go like this (Mr. Vanguard's responses are in italics):

What is the name of the case?

Cocaine Kid

What does the therapist think the problem is?

cocaine abuse

Would the client agree that this is the problem?

y

Has someone already started doing something, i.e., is there DELIBERATE presession change?

y

Does this change seem rapid?

y

Do they know what they need to do to keep these behaviors which are involved in the presession change going?

n

Are they confident about keeping it going?

n

*   *   *

Was the therapist able to get the client to follow nonverbal leads?

y

Are other individuals contributing to the problem?

y

Is someone necessary to the solution absent from this session?

n

* * *

Pardon me while I think about this case. . . .

rule 111 suggests: give a task to do more of what they are doing

rule 113 suggests: give task to notice what is different about those occasions when they keep change going

rule 589 suggests: consider giving a task that interrupts the way in which others contribute to the client's problem

Based upon the advice given by BRIEFER, and his own clinical observations during the interview, Mr. Vanguard designs a task which he then assigns to his client. In addition to advising Ms. Jones to continue unplugging the phone, knitting, etc., Mr. Vanguard also asks that she get her parents to sign a statement that they will never again loan her the money to buy drugs. Mr. Vanguard then concludes the session, after scheduling a return appointment.

Although BRIEFER is currently only a demonstration prototype, with further development and testing it should be able to give useful advice to beginning therapists.

WHAT ARE EXPERT SYSTEMS?

Expert systems are computer programs which are designed to embody the expertise of a human expert in order to consult on a specific problem. In practice an expert system works much like a human consultant — the computer asks the user a series of questions about the specific problem, then it processes the information it has received, and then it offers advice. If it is a fully-developed expert system, the advice it gives may equal or surpass that given by human experts.

Expert systems comprise one subfield within the larger field of artificial intelligence. Artificial intelligence is an interdisciplinary field concerned with developing computer programs that behave in ways normally associated with human intelligence (Schuerman, in press). Expert systems comprise a relatively new area; the first expert systems were developed in the 1970s in the AI labs at Stanford University, MIT and Carnegie-Mellon. The technology has developed very rapidly, however, with the first commercial expert systems appearing in the late 1970s and early 1980s. Full utilization of the technology is still a few years off, when easy to use tools will be widely available at a reasonable cost.

Prior to the advent of artificial intelligence and expert systems, computers were limited to straightforward data processing applications. Problems had to be quantifiable and subject to algorithmic solution for computers to be useful (Schoech, Jennings, Schkade and Hooper-Russell, 1985). That is, if the problem could be reduced to numbers, and a precise formula for its solution could be identified, the computer could be programmed to produce the solution. Examples of such conventional data processing applications are accounting and statistical programs, and most database management programs. Although the data processing approach has proven very useful for administrative and financial management functions, it has not found widespread application in the day to day work of most human service practitioners. Much of human service work, by its very nature, cannot be quantified and reduced to algorithmic solutions.

Expert systems technology may change that, however. This new technology provides a useful way to apply the tremendous computing power of modern, high speed, and relatively inexpensive computers to the ill-defined but important practical problems in the human services.

Expert systems are distinguished from conventional programs by the fact that they manipulate symbolic data rather than quantitative data (Waterman, 1986). Further, expert systems use heuristics (rules of thumb) rather than algorithms to solve problems. Finally, expert systems are able to use inference or reasoning to reach conclusions. Some expert systems can even examine their own reasoning, and explain their operation to the user. These characteristics make it possible for expert systems to solve "ill defined" problems that may be idiosyncratic, and about which there may be incomplete information.

Just as there are many kinds of human expertise, there are many kinds of expert systems. Most expert systems are best characterized as diagnostic or prescriptive, or both. Medical expert systems diagnose illnesses and prescribe drug therapy or other treatment. In industry, expert systems diagnose malfunctions of complex machines and prescribe the steps necessary to repair them. Other expert systems plan or design complex activities such as how to configure a new computer system, or how to synthesize new molecules. Still other expert systems monitor and control nuclear reactors or patients' reactions to drug regimens.

The earliest and best known expert systems were developed in the area of medical practice. Probably the most famous is MYCIN, an expert system designed to aid physicians in the diagnosis and treatment of meningitis and bacteremia infections (Buchanan & Shortliffe, 1984). MYCIN was developed at Stanford University in the 1970s and was the first large expert system to perform at the level of a human expert (Harmon & King, 1985). To use MYCIN, the physician sits in front of a computer terminal and answers a series of questions. MYCIN asks about characteristics of the patient, symptoms, and lab test results. If the physician doesn't know the answer to a question, MYCIN will reason with incomplete information. The physician may also indicate a degree of uncertainty when answering. All of these features enable MYCIN to perform much like a human consultant. MYCIN first diagnoses the problem, then after additional interaction with the physician recommends a course of treatment for the patient. If the physician wants to know how MYCIN reached its conclusions, MYCIN will provide its rationale.

Although many medical expert systems have been developed to date, several are of particular interest. INTERNIST, and its later version CADUCEUS, are some of the largest medical expert systems developed to date, containing profiles of more than 500 diseases (Miller, Pople and Myers, 1982). CADUCEUS has reportedly passed the diagnostic portion of the Board Certification exam for internal medicine (Schoech et al., 1985). It is expected that CADUCEUS will eventually be available to practicing physicians on a time-share basis for use in diagnosing difficult cases.

One of the few expert systems having to do with psychological functioning is BLUE BOX, which advises physicians on selecting therapy for depressed patients (Mulsant and Servan-Schreiber, 1984). BLUE BOX was developed using EMYCIN ("Empty"

MYCIN), the expert system inference engine which was developed in the MYCIN project.

GUIDON is an expert system which uses the knowledge base and case examples in MYCIN to tutor physicians in training (Clancey, 1983). GUIDON selects one of its patients for the student to consider and then solves the problem just as MYCIN would. Having done so, GUIDON then invites the student to ask questions, much as MYCIN asks the physician questions. GUIDON follows the student's questioning (and diagnostic logic) and if it finds the student is asking irrelevant questions or gets off the track, it provides corrective explanations. Although GUIDON has not proven completely satisfactory as a tutoring device, it is an interesting attempt to make explicit use of the knowledge contained in an expert system for use in professional training.

A number of expert systems are currently under development in the fields of education and social services. A group at the University of Texas at Arlington is developing an expert system which will advise on whether a person with a disability is a good candidate for more detailed screening by a technology specialist (Dick Schoech, personal communication, January, 1986). Schuerman (1986) at the University of Chicago has developed PLACECON, an experimental expert system designed to advise on child placement in child welfare practice. A group in England is working on expert systems to assist in the management of enuresis (Toole, Harvey & Winfield, 1987). Educational researchers at Utah State University have developed Class.LD2 for classifying learning disabled students (Ferrara & Hofmeister, 1984), and Behavior Consultant for advising on data collection procedures and intervention strategies for child behavior problems in the classroom (Ferrara, Serna & Baer, 1986). Mental health researchers at the Missouri Institute of Psychiatry have developed CATCEC, an expert system to assist non-mental-health-experts in treating emotional emergencies (Hedlund, Vieweg and Cho, 1987). A group at the University of Wisconsin-Milwaukee and the Brief Family Therapy Center have developed BRIEFER, a demonstration prototype expert system which advises the brief family therapist on intervention design (Goodman, 1986; Goodman, Gingerich & de Shazer, 1987). Most of these systems are still in the development and testing phases, but they indicate the types of applications that expert systems will likely be addressing in the near future.

WHY USE AN EXPERT SYSTEM?

There are a number of important reasons why expert systems technology has potential value in day to day practice. Real human expertise, like the expertise embodied in an experienced and highly trained internist, is usually in short supply. Human experts cannot easily be reproduced and distributed; human expertise is the result of long and specialized training and many years of experience. Computer expert systems, however, can be copied and distributed very easily and inexpensively, making expertise widely available to many.

Human expertise is also quite perishable, that is, it can be lost quickly through disuse, employee turnover, or death. Computerized expertise, since it is saved on magnetic tape or disk, is permanent.

Computer expertise may also be more reliable and consistent than human expertise. Human experts are influenced by many physical and psychological factors when they make decisions, resulting in a certain degree of unreliability. Several evaluations have shown that not only are computer expert systems sometimes more valid than human experts, but that recognized human experts often do not agree among themselves (Yu et al., 1984; Martindale, Ferrara and Campbell, 1986).

PROMISE AND PITFALLS

Pitfalls

As with any new technology, although expert systems hold considerable promise for human services practice they are not a panacea.

Costly to build. While it is possible to get a prototype expert system up and running within several months, the development and evaluation necessary to develop a full working expert system require considerable resources in time and money. Some human service problems probably justify such an expenditure (e.g., determining risk of child abuse or neglect) whereas others do not.

Limited applications. Given the current state of the art, expert systems appear to be limited to a fairly narrow range of human service problems, mainly diagnosing and prescribing types of activities. Further, the problems must be ones for which genuine human expertise exists, that is, recognized experts agree on the solution. Given the lack of precise knowledge that characterizes many human service problems, the range of possible applications is restricted.

Limitations of the technology. At their current level of development, expert systems are not very good at knowing their own limitations, and they are not proficient at common sense reasoning. Thus, expert systems are appropriate only for problems for which the relevant parameters are clearly established. Expert systems also are not able to acquire or update their knowledge base as human experts do, so they require continual updating and elaboration, particularly in fields in which the knowledge and practice is still evolving. If knowledge about a problem is changing too rapidly, it is not a good candidate for an expert system. Expert systems also cannot evaluate their own knowledge to identify gaps or inconsistencies. Expert systems are still "dumb" systems in the sense that they have very limited capacity to learn from experience.

Ethical issues. As Schoech et al. (1986) have noted, the use of expert systems in human services practice raises some ethical issues. For example, must a practitioner consult an expert system if one is available? Must the advice it gives be followed? What is the liability of the developer of the expert system? Legal and ethical guidelines for these and other issues have yet to be established, but for the present time the practitioner should certainly not suspend his or her judgment to follow blindly the advice of the expert system, even though the expert system has been thoroughly evaluated. Expert systems should be considered aids to the professional's decision-making, not substitutes for it.

Promise

Support of professional decision-making. The most direct benefit to be derived from expert systems is the improvement in professional decision-making which they may provide. Expertise in human services is frequently in short supply and spread too thin. If an expert system can be made to perform at a level equal to the best human experts, then the best advice will be available to all professionals.

Expert systems technology may also facilitate the dissemination of new knowledge. As knowledge in a problem domain changes it can be reflected in updates to the expert system, which in turn can easily be distributed to all users. This requires ongoing support and maintenance of the expert system, but resources invested in this way will likely have a larger and more immediate impact than efforts to retrain practicing professionals in the problem domain. Of course, expert systems technology should never be thought of as a substitute for professional training and professional judgment. It will increasingly become an important means of support to professional decision-making, however.

Training. Expert systems which incorporate good explanation and help facilities can provide limited training for the practicing professional. This is particularly true for professionals in training. As users interact with the expert system, they learn what pieces of information are relevant to the problem, and what the appropriate decision rules are. Further, as technology develops, it may be possible to use the knowledge bases developed for expert systems to directly tutor students (Clancey, 1983).

Description and codification of knowledge. Perhaps one of the most interesting and useful side benefits of expert systems is their contribution to the development and codification of professional knowledge. Because human experts frequently find it difficult to elucidate their problem-solving knowledge, much of the knowledge derived from practice is probably never adequately described or passed on. The knowledge acquisition and representation process for building an expert system almost always results in significant advances in the description and codification of professional knowledge. Some might argue that this side benefit alone justifies the development of expert systems. As knowledge engineering techniques improve, we can expect to see even more benefits in the description and codification of professional knowledge.

What the future may hold. Because expert systems technology is still very new it is difficult to anticipate the kinds of applications and benefits we may realize in the future. Some directions seem to be emerging, however. Expert systems technology will be applied to increasingly large and complex problems. Until now, expert systems have generally been limited to small, narrow problems which a single human expert could solve. But the nature of many important problems is that they are interdisciplinary, requiring perhaps more expertise than a single human being can possess. As the technology improves, we may begin to see the development of expert systems which are more competent than humans at solving such complex problems. This is most likely to occur where decisions require the continuous monitoring of large amounts of information, or where many detailed and interdependent rules are required for reaching decisions.

It is likely that as the technology develops we will see expert systems that do more than diagnose and prescribe treatment. Expert systems may assist professionals in case management, intervention and program design, and perhaps even clinical assessment, interviewing and report writing.

Some day expert systems may have the capacity to examine their own reasoning systems and knowledge bases, and in the process begin to develop new knowledge themselves. While computers may never be very creative in the usual sense, they may be able to perform some intelligent activities having to do with the synthesis and analysis of information.

It is clear that expert systems technology will have increasing importance for human service practice, inasmuch as it provides a way of applying the tremendous information processing capacity of modern computers to the knowledge based activities of the practicing professional. Although care must continually be exercised to insure that the technology is not used inappropriately or inadvisedly, human service professionals should actively pursue creative applications of expert systems technology for the betterment of the profession and the clients they serve.

REFERENCES

Buchanan, B. G., & Shortliffe, E. H. (Eds.). (1984). *Rule-based expert systems*. Reading, MA: Addison-Wesley.
Clancey, W. J. (1983). GUIDON. *Journal of Computer-Based Instruction, 10* (1 & 2), 8-15.

de Shazer, S. (1985). *Keys to solution in brief therapy*. New York: W. W. Norton.

de Shazer, S., Berg, I. K., Lipchik, E., Nunnally, E., Molnar, A., Gingerich, W., & Weiner-Davis, M. (1986). Brief therapy: Focused solution development. *Family Process, 25*, 207-221.

Ferrara, J. M., & Hofmeister, A. M. (1984). *Class.LD2: An expert system for classifying learning disabilities* [Computer program]. Logan, UT: Utah State University, Artificial Intelligence Research and Development Unit, Developmental Center for Handicapped Persons.

Ferrara, J. M., Serna, R. W., & Baer, R. D. (1986). *Behavior consultant: An expert system for the diagnosis of social/emotional behavioral problems* [Computer program]. Logan, UT: Utah State University, Artificial Intelligence Research and Development Unit, Developmental Center for Handicapped Persons.

Goodman, H. (1986). *BRIEFER: An expert system for brief family therapy*. Unpublished master's thesis, University of Wisconsin-Milwaukee, Milwaukee, WI.

Goodman, H., Gingerich, W. J., & de Shazer, S. (1987). *BRIEFER: An expert system for clinical practice*. Manuscript submitted for publication.

Harmon, P. & King, D. (1985). *Expert systems*. New York: John Wiley & Sons.

Hedlund, J. L., Vieweg, B. W., & Cho, D. W. (1987). *Computer consultation for emotional crises: an expert system for "non-experts."* St. Louis: Missouri Institute of Psychiatry.

Martindale, E. S., Ferrara, J. M., & Campbell, B. W. (1986). *Accuracy of Class.LD2: An expert system for classifying learning disabled students*. Unpublished manuscript, Utah State University, Department of Special Education.

Miller, R. A., Pople, Jr., H. E., & Myers, J. D. (1982). INTERNIST-I, an experimental computer-based diagnostic consultant for general internal medicine. *New England Journal of Medicine, 307*, 468-476.

Mulsant, B. & Servan-Schreiber, D. (1984). Knowledge engineering: A daily activity on a hospital ward. *Computers and Biomedical Research, 17*, 71-91.

Schoech, D., Jennings, H., Schkade, L. L., & Hooper-Russell, C. (1985). Expert systems: Artificial intelligence for professional decisions. *Computers in Human Services, 1*, 81-115.

Schuerman, J. R. (1986). *PLACECON* [Computer program]. Chicago: University of Chicago, School of Social Service Administration.

Schuerman, J. R. (in press). Expert consulting systems in social welfare. *Social Work Research and Abstracts*.

Toole, S. K., Harvey, C. K., & Winfield, M. J. (1987). *An assessment of expert systems techniques for the human services*. Birmingham, England: Birmingham Polytechnic Expert Systems Group.

Weiner-Davis, M., de Shazer, S. & Gingerich, W. (in press). Using pretreatment change to construct a therapeutic solution: A clinical note. *Journal of Marital and Family Therapy*.

Waterman, D. A. (1986). *A guide to expert systems*. Reading, MA: Addison-Wesley.

Yu, V. L., Fagan, L. M., Bennett, S. W., Clancey, W. J., Scott, A. C., Hannigan, J. F., Blum, R. L., Buchanan, B. G., & Cohen, S. N. (1984). An evaluation of MYCIN's advice. In B. G. Buchanan and E. H. Shortliffe (Eds.), *Rule-based expert systems* (pp. 589-596). New York: Addison-Wesley.

Computer Assisted Decision Making

Elizabeth Mutschler

KEYWORDS. Computers, decision support system, expert system, information system, clinical decision making, decision theory

SUMMARY. It is frequently argued that computerized decision support lends itself more easily to structured than to semi- or unstructured decisions. This paper discusses decision tasks of human service practitioners and surveys emerging research in decision theory and associated decision applications. It provides examples of an Information System, a Decision Support, and an Expert System, and examines under what conditions they can facilitate decision making in human services. A number of future issues and concerns are addressed, including ethical and legal questions, and computer literacy in human services education and practice.

INTRODUCTION

Human service activities can be viewed within a decision making framework, in recognition of the many decisions practitioners have to make and help others make (Gambrill & Stein, 1983). The computer can support the practitioners' decision tasks through its inexhaustible capacities for routine information processing, its vast memory banks, and its rapid, accurate, and consistent data retrieval capabilities. Recent interdisciplinary research combining decision theory and information technology offers great potential to aid the

Elizabeth Mutschler, PhD, is Associate Professor at the School of Social Work, The University of Michigan, Ann Arbor, MI. She has published extensively on subjects of evaluation research, research utilization, the development of information systems and their applications in social work practice and education. She is currently involved in a study developing decision support systems for clinical practice in human service agencies.

231

decision tasks of practitioners, but the actual use of computerized decision tools — especially in clinical practice — has been limited and slow to develop. This paper (1) presents a decision making framework for analyzing human service activities; (2) describes how information, decision support, and expert systems can contribute to human service decision making; and (3) discusses issues and future developments related to computerized decision applications in human services. This discussion is by necessity brief and incomplete, but it and the accompanying reference list may help the interested reader who wishes to learn more about the emerging field of computerized decision applications in human service organizations.

A DECISION FRAMEWORK: CONCEPTS AND DEFINITIONS

The tasks of human service practitioners can be described on a continuum from structured, semi-structured, to unstructured decisions. The concept of task or decision structure has been developed by Keen and Morton (1978) based on Simon's early distinction between programmed and non-programmed decisions (1960). Structured tasks are generally repetitive and routine, with established and well-explicated procedures. Semi- or unstructured decisions may be made at irregular intervals and tend to be confronted anew each time they arise due to their complexity. Data items guiding unstructured decisions and the way these items are combined vary from decision to decision (Keen and Morton, 1978); decision processes are heuristic rather than prescribed.

Structured tasks, where procedures are clearly specified, include business applications such as accounting, billing, personnel monitoring, as well as simple administrative and case management systems. Routinely used forms are already a component of the manual operation, and the flow of data is well defined. Client interviews and selected diagnostic assessment procedures are examples of semi-structured tasks. Previous work has shown that if assessment and diagnostic procedures can be explicated carefully, it is then possible to develop software to administer, score, and interpret computerized client interviews accurately and reliably (Greist et al., 1980; Slack et al., 1977). Examples of unstructured decisions include tasks related to treatment planning, monitoring, and implementation. In spite of the complexity of unstructured tasks, expert practitioners do somehow manage to meet a new client or family, ask a number of questions, arrive at a treatment plan subject to future adjustment, and arrange their information gathering and intervention strategies accordingly. Buchanan (1984) notes that this view of semi- and unstructured decision tasks involves the selection of a leading subset of hypotheses from "a world of hypotheses" that may number dozens or even hundreds. The practitioner's strategy of collecting additional information guided by an initial set of hypotheses often allows client and clinician during the first intake interview(s) to generate both a preliminary set of treatment objectives and a plan of action. This fascinating and elusive process is increasingly a subject of study. A better understanding of how expert practitioners generate and refine hypotheses regarding treatment objectives, interventions, and related outcomes, will help us to provide design criteria for programs that can effectively assist in the assessment and treatment of semi- and unstructured client problem situations.

DECISION APPLICATIONS IN HUMAN SERVICE AGENCIES

To illustrate how computer applications can assist human service professionals in their decision making, examples of three types of computer systems will be described: Information Systems (IS), Decision Support Systems (DSS), and Expert Systems (ES).

Information Systems (IS)

One of the most typical ways of introducing computers into human service agencies is through the development of a basic information system aimed at improving the efficiency of routine decision tasks. As was described earlier, structured decision tasks are generally repetitive and routine, with established and clearly defined procedures. An information system consists of sets of logically related data files, or data bases and an associated grouping of software (programs) necessary to store, manage, and retrieve data from the data base. The availability of small microcomputers with rapid response time and inexpensive on-line access to information has resulted in an increased interest and use of information systems by human service agencies (Mutschler, 1986; Hedlund et al., 1985). A prototype of an integrated clinical and fiscal information system for small to medium-sized human service agencies was developed at Gateway Children's Society (Mutschler and Hasenfeld, 1985). Gateway Children's Society provides residential care for about 50 children with behavioral problems. It also has a day treatment program for 120 children, and a small adoption and foster care program. Smaller agencies usually have less access to information technology resources, consultants, and programmers. The purpose of the project was to develop a model information system, general and flexible enough to be applied in other small to medium-sized non-profit agencies. A key principle in the successful development of this information system was to compile available data in ways that were meaningful to staff members communicating information to them for their day-to-day decisions. The system's objectives were to:

1. document the flow of clients and the provision of services
2. give immediate feedback to direct service providers and keep records current
3. meet internal and external reporting needs for data on clients and services
4. meet financial reporting requirements for funding sources and provide a data base for fiscal review
5. provide summary information for client and agency management, and
6. be able to perform cost-outcome analysis.

One requirement of the computerized information system was to convert the previously used manual recording system into a series of standardized input forms. These forms then captured specific client and service information critical to the practitioners' decisions at major treatment junctures. All levels of staff were involved in designing the new recording system, and the required internal and external reports, to insure their applicability to the staff's day-to-day tasks.

The client-based part of the information system represents mainly a client-tracking mechanism. It provides information for routine case management tasks and decisions such as assessing how many new clients to accept into the program, monitoring caseloads of line workers, preparing intake and discharge reports for clients, and obtaining summary reports about workers' caseloads. The worker is also able to obtain descriptive information about clients relating to services provided, or family characteristics, useful for the planning and implementation of treatment and for the eventual discharge planning.

The next phase of the project involves the expansion of the basic information system to include data for decision tasks more directly related to treatment implementation and evaluation. Representing mostly semi-structured decisions, this phase of the project is currently being developed. For example, a task force has designed a computerized behavioral monitoring instrument for clients in the residential treatment program which identifies target behaviors, and allows staff to monitor client functioning over time. This instrument provides critical information for treatment planning, monitoring and evaluation, and for the planning of discharge.

As can be seen in this example the strength of an information system is to efficiently collect, store, and process a large amount of data. ISs can support stuctured, semi-structured, and potentially also unstructured decisions. One difference between structured and semi-structured decisions in the described IS was the effort required to identify decision criteria and the information needed for specific tasks. For example, the procedures and criteria for accepting a new case in the residential program were relatively well-established and defined (i.e., a structured decision task). The information needed for the placement decision could therefore be identified and incorporated into the IS with relatively little effort.

The criteria for deciding when a resident was "ready for discharge" seemed to be more complex. Criteria guiding the discharge decision and the way these decision criteria were combined frequently varied from worker to worker and from case to case, thus representing a semi-structured task. The computerized behavior monitoring instrument, developed by a task force over a period of several months, provided the basis for identifying discharge criteria related to client functioning.

Users have to identify, therefore, which decision tasks are most likely to be amenable to a computerized information system. As has been shown in this example, semi- or unstructured decisions can be codified and can be incorporated successfully into an IS. Conversely, not every structured decision is automatically suitable for a computerized IS. We recently considered whether or not to include computerized information for deciding whether to refer a client to group therapy (as compared to individual therapy). After we identified the decision criteria, we found out that the potential client pool for group therapy was very small. We decided therefore it would not be cost-effective to include information for group placement in the IS. A professional could collect this information and make that decision more efficiently at intake. Thus, for each decision area users should weigh the costs of developing a computerized IS in relation to the benefits that will be obtained.

In contrast to ISs, decision support systems go beyond the collection and retrieval of information. They are aimed at enhancing the effectiveness of decision makers. The next section describes an example of a decision support system successfully used in a Home Supportive Services Program.

Decision Support Systems (DSS)

The concept of decision support systems was first articulated by Scott Morton in the early 70s (Scott Morton, 1971). DSSs are interactive computer support systems designed to enhance the effectiveness of decision makers in organizations (Vogel, 1985). Since DSSs are frequently defined in such general terms, the concept is often used as an umbrella term encompassing a wide range of computer systems that facilitate decision making. Vogel provides a list of more specific DSS characteristics:

1. DSSs are intended to be supportive to decision makers, not to replace them;
2. DSSs are aimed at less well-structured problems which tend to lack complete specification;

3. DSSs seek to combine the use of models and analytic techniques with more customary data access and retrieval functions;

4. DSSs are interactive and "friendly" to the decision maker, and are therefore supportive to users who are not computer specialists;

5. DSSs are intentionally flexible in order to adapt to changes in the organization's environment and to the individual needs of the decision makers;

6. DSSs often involve the use of large data bases whose structure and content may be overwhelming to the decision maker in the absence of supportive tools (Vogel, 1985, p. 68).

At the highest level of DSS technology the system incorporates the decision context whose dimensions include the tasks and problem setting, user's skills and previous decisions, and the organizational environment (Bennett, 1983). A DSS can provide the user with an enhanced support to execute decision tasks, to easily manipulate model structures, or to query data bases.

A DSS successfully used in a Home Supportive Services Program in California has been reported by Boyd et al. (1982). The Home Supportive Services Program (HSS) serves approximately 80,000 elderly disabled clients at an annual cost approaching one-quarter of a billion dollars. Based on a legally prescribed home visit, the 120 line workers make two decisions about the client. First, the client's degree of need (an assessment decision), and second, the worker determines the weekly hours of service the client should receive (a distribution decision). According to the report, the distribution of HSS services was marked by inequality. In place of a common standard, each worker more or less created his or her own. Since the workers treated the collective wisdom of their peers as more authoritative than state or county regulations, an attempt was made to improve equity through a DSS which would inform the discretionary behavior of line workers, supervisors and managers.

Each HSS district received a microcomputer which tabulated the average number of hours all workers would award to a specific type of client. Workers then developed a set of quantitative client needs scales by identifying which client characteristics influence their award decisions. These scales were used to identify workers' decision rules. This initial process sparked sufficient dialogue among workers to yield an agreed-upon first edition of a standardized assessment form, which facilitated the entry of cases into the microcomputer. As assessments became more reliable, it became possible to analyze workers' distribution decisions to discover the implicit weights workers gave to different client characteristics in determining client awards. This analysis resulted in a distributive formula or algorithm which, once entered into the computer, would convert a worker's assessment of a client into a predicted award. Given the distributive rule formula, it became possible to report how much a worker's judgment strayed from current collective wisdom. Should a worker's award be substantially higher or lower than predicted, the worker was prompted for a comment on the uniqueness of that case. For example, the comment "must see doctor three times a week and no public transportation is available" is entered into and stored in the computer. Through successive approximations and workers' feedback, assessment forms and computer programs were revised and a refined distributive formula was entered into the program. Reports were developed that told each worker how the pattern of his/her assessment and distribution decisions compared to the pattern of his/her unit and county. Various aggregations of worker reports were prepared for supervisors and managers.

At the beginning of the project approximately 60% of the variance in client awards was explained by client characteristics. Two years after the implementation of the DSS, that variance was up to 85% and was still rising. Thus, for the first time, the DSS provided 120 workers in the three demonstration counties with information that discretionary decisions required. Once so informed, equity increased while less administrative control and fewer top-down rules were needed (Boyd et al., 1982). Thus the DSS not only provided needed information to practitioners, but also improved the quality of their decision making.

This example illustrates a number of the DSS characteristics identified by Vogel (1985): the lineworkers were the ultimate decision makers since they could accept or reject (based on professional reasoning) the decisions of the computerized DSS. At the same time, the DSS was flexible enough to adapt to individual needs of clients and to changes in their environment. Once the components of the assessment and the distribution decision were identified, a distributive formula or algorithm could be developed which facilitated standardization and equity of the lineworkers' decisions, thereby improving not only efficiency but also the effectiveness of their work. Without the computerized DSS, keeping track of the entire data base of elderly disabled clients, and coordinating lineworkers' decisions for these clients would have been almost impossible. Finally, the DSS was interactive and "friendly" to the lineworker and required minimum training for users who were not computer specialists.

Expert Systems (ES)

Expert Systems are one of a number of recent developments that provide support for human service decision making. Expert systems are computer programs which use inference schemes to apply generalized human expertise to the facts of a specific case (Schoech et al., 1985). ESs have evolved from a field of study called "Artificial Intelligence" (AI), which is concerned with giving computing systems the capabilities normally associated with human intelligence such as reasoning, learning, and self-improvement (Schoech et al., 1985). One of the subfields of applied AI is concerned with the development of systems which embody the knowledge of experts in particular areas. Such systems are called "Expert Systems," "Consultation Systems," or "Knowledge Based Systems." Thus, an expert system can infer knowledge and make recommendations based upon facts and rules that go far beyond the information stored in the data base. Decision tasks amenable to the development of an expert system are usually non-routine, require reasoning about the facts of a given situation, exercise some judgment, and require professional skill and knowledge.

In general, expert systems consist of three parts: (1) an inference mechanism, (2) a knowledge base associated with decision rules, and (3) a set of facts (or a data base). The inference mechanism applies rules to facts and thereby generates new facts and recommendations. This component of the ES assumes that complex decision tasks can be broken down into concrete decisions that can be represented in the form of if-then rules. The inference mechanism has control functions that determine under what conditions which rules should be applied to which facts; it also provides the "interface" with the user. That is, it asks questions of the user and reports conclusions. A major part of developing an ES consists of working with experts and professionals in specific knowledge areas to uncover the rules underlying their decisions (Schuerman, 1986).

The rules in an expert system thus embody specific knowledge of a particular domain. They typically indicate how strongly a given inference can be drawn when specific observations are made. An example of a rule from an experimental consulting system for child placement is:

IF: Placement is needed, and   )
        Relatives are available to care for the child, and   )   Premise
        Relatives are willing,   )
THEN: PLACE THE CHILD WITH RELATIVES   Conclusion
        (Schuerman, 1986)

This example illustrates the form of a typical rule used in an ES. The premise is the conditional portion of the rule and is formed by the conjunction of a set of conditions, all of which must be true for the rule to hold. When the premises of a rule are true there is reason to believe that its conclusion is true.

As described by Schuerman (1986), the third component of an expert system refers to the facts of a specific situation. In clinical practice it is usually a particular client case. Facts such as family or problem characteristics will be different for each case. Since the ES may be consulted at various points in the life of a client, the facts can change even for the same case.

Some ESs have the capability to deal with uncertainty by attaching probability values or uncertainty factors to facts and rules. For example, if it is almost certain that relatives are willing and able to care for the child, the probability would be .95; if it is questionable, the probability might be .60. The inference mechanism combines the certainty values of all facts and rules to determine the certainty (or probability) of the conclusion or recommendation generated by the system. To summarize, an expert system can be defined as consisting of a knowledge base associated with decision rules, and an inference mechanism that is triggered by the practitioner's input of specific facts about clients and/or their problem situations.

The human services field is still in its early stages of developing and testing applications of expert systems. An example is the earlier mentioned ES developed by Schuerman (1986), which makes recommendations on the placement of children in child welfare practice. The ES is written in a language called LISP and is named PLACECON. While the system is still in its experimental stage and is not to be used in routine practice, it delineates clearly the required tasks and procedures in the development of an expert system. The program asks a series of questions about the child, the family, available placement options, and then reports recommendations as to what type of placement or services are indicated in this case. A particular strength of this program is its explanation capability. For example, when the user asks "Why" or "How" a certain recommendation was deduced, the program can report the rules, facts, and the probabilities assigned to each that led to the particular conclusion. This is a very useful feature. It allows the user to examine the appropriateness of the rules, points out which rules need to be revised, and what additional rules might be needed.

Schoech et al. (1985) developed a similar rule-based expert system written in BASIC. The system determines the priority of a new abuse case during the child abuse investigation by a public child welfare agency. The experimental program is using thirteen rules to establish one of four hypotheses. For example, "the case is priority one," indicating very serious abuse and a high need for protection, or "the case is priority three," indicating less serious abuse and low need for protection. An excerpt from an expert system session illustrates the user-computer interchange. The user can answer the program's questions with Y (Yes), N (No), or W (why). If the user responds with W, the program displays the rule(s) and fact(s) applied in drawing a conclusion.

Is it true: Burns exist on child? N
Is it true: Child has broken bones? N
Is it true: Discipline is excessive? W
I am trying to use rule 1.

If: Discipline is excessive,
  No physical injury exists from discipline
Then: Abuse not serious.
Is it true: Discipline is excessive? Y
Is it true: No physical injury exists from discipline? Y
Rule 1 deduces: Abuse not serious.
Rule 10 deduces: Case is priority 2. (Schoech et al., p. 93)

Combined with the computer's capacity for rapid, accurate and consistent data processing, an expert system is a powerful tool for human service practitioners. But we have to be aware that the judgment and inferential ability of an ES is totally limited by the knowledge base and the rules that are used in generating the information and recommendations. A number of issues need to be addressed, therefore, as ESs are being developed and introduced into direct practice. What level of computer literacy and knowledge about information technology must human service professionals have in order to become active participants and innovators of change? What skills and information do they need to insure that emerging decision tools and technology will be responsive to the complex needs of social work practitioners? How well is the theory and practice of social work intervention proceduralized? Do we know enough about the rules social workers use in arriving at their decisions? And finally, who decides what is acceptable knowledge, practice, and policy?

As the profession increases its knowledge of decision applications, the potential as well as the limitations of these applications become apparent. The development of decision tools becomes at once exciting and complex, challenging and diverse. Some of the described issues, as well as potential future directions in the development and application of information technology in the human services will be addressed in the next section.

ISSUES AND IMPLICATIONS

This review illustrates that Human Service Agencies have the greatest experience with the application of information systems. ISs can improve the efficiency of decision making and are used mostly for structured decision tasks (Mutschler, 1986; Hedlund et al., 1985). Computer support for semi-structured and unstructured decisions in human services is emerging but still needs additional research and development. Expert systems have a number of potential applications. They provide feedback or suggested courses of action. They also can advance a practitioner's level of expertise by defining or clarifying the knowledge base and inference processes professionals use in their decision. As Schoech points out, expert systems may also be used to assist novice workers in locations where human service resources are scarce, such as in rural areas or overcrowded and understaffed practice settings (Schoech et al., 1985). However, in order to make computer applications responsive to complex decision tasks, particularly in clinical practice, a number of issues need to be addressed.

Knowledge Base and Decision Rules

As we examine the type and level of computer abilities needed to successfully use information technology in human services, it becomes evident that many of the fundamental issues are related more to the state of knowledge about decision processes and decision support than to technical issues related to computer hardware and software. The productive use of expert systems is unlikely to occur until we are able to describe the actual decision making processes that take place in the human services. More knowledge, for example, about decision structures and the rules decision makers use, and more data are needed on the wide range of decisions that exist in the human services. We also need to know how the decision structures differ by organizational level, types of services or interventions used, the nature of the problem, or the particular role played by the decision maker. It is likely that the most useful outcome of efforts to build expert systems will not be in the finished product, but rather in the codification and systematization of knowledge within the field. In developing decision tools, the interrelationships of principles must be explicated and inconsistencies and contradictions ferreted out. The development process also helps in identifying gaps in knowledge; it makes assumptions explicit enough to be recognized and challenged. In addition, the DSS example, reveals, how with the codification of knowledge will come a concomitant standardization of practice (Boyd et al., 1982). Since successful expert systems contain a substantial body of knowledge, they may also prove to be a helpful learning tool. As mentioned earlier, novice social workers or students can then learn about general principles embodied in the decision rules, what information needs to be collected, and how to determine when unique client situations require exceptions to normally operating rules (Lynett, 1986; Schuerman, 1987).

Selecting Computerized Decision Applications

Users need to distinguish between decision tasks that require an information system, a decision support system, or an expert system. The examples in this paper illustrating each type of decision application do not imply that an expert system is always appropriate for unstructured decisions or an information system for structured decision tasks. If the complexities of a semi-structured task can be explicated and codified, a sophisticated client information system may be more cost-effective and more appropriate than a DSS or an ES. If we can encode data items and related decision processes in the form of an algorithm, a decision support system might be appropriate. Algorithm-based DSSs are most effective if we can codify a frequently used decision function such as allocating working hours of home support services, or determining eligibility for financial aid. If the decision tasks involve learning about decision rules and decision processes, flexibility of and adaptation to semi- or unstructured tasks, or the evolution of potentially new decision functions, then an expert system might be appropriate. An area is usually considered a candidate for the development of expert systems if it requires reasoning about the facts of a given situation, followed by the exercise of some judgment in an area requiring professional skill and knowledge. Often the judgments to be made are based on processes which the human expert cannot fully specify. On the other hand, however, areas characterized by a great deal of novelty or by a need for real creativity, that is, completely unstructured decisions, are unlikely to yield to an expert system approach (Schuerman, 1987). Users should also be aware that various models of ESs are being developed and tested experimentally. Very few, if any, ESs are currently used on a routine basis in human service agencies.

Initial Focus Should Be on Limited Scope of Decision Tasks

Upon closer scrutiny of the described decision support and expert systems we find that they involve a relatively small number of decisions. While the DSS focuses on generating the weekly hours of home-based services, the expert system specifies the type of placement in child welfare, or the priority of a child abuse case. In situations where there is a large domain of potential decisions, such as diagnoses and treatment recommendations in family therapy, it may be more difficult to develop an effective expert system. Bennett (1983) recommends, for example, starting with a limited scope of the system sufficient to satisfy the user need for support. For example, rather than developing an expert system for a family agency that includes diagnosis, treatment planning and implementation, start with a system that incorporates knowledge and decision rules related to intake only.

Interactive Nature of Decision Applications

Decision applications usually generate learning and new insights, but they also stimulate new uses and the need for new functions in the system. Decision applications are thus shaped by and in turn shape the context in which they evolve. For example, when practitioners attempt to identify their decision rules, they frequently discover that their actual criteria are different from the ones they thought they were applying (Boyd et al., 1982). Decision applications are therefore more likely to be used if practitioners are able to take into account the evolving decision context whose dimensions include the task or problem setting, the user's preferences and skills, the procedures and rules for decision making, and the organizational environment (Bennett, 1983).

FUTURE DEVELOPMENT

Many writers in the field agree with Henderson (1986) that the choice not to use computers is not available to human service organizations. If the professionals in the field ignore the available information systems, others outside of the field will impose the technology. The issue for human service professionals is therefore to become as knowledgeable and informed as possible about the potential, as well as the limitations or negative consequences of the use of information technology. Professionals also need to participate in the ethical and legal decisions that have to be made as to the conditions under which such technologies can or cannot be applied.

Ethical and Legal Questions

At a recent conference on information technology in human services, a "CODE OF ETHICS" regarding values and ethics in relation to technological applications in the human services was proposed. In its summary paragraph, it states:

> We wish to affirm our commitment to the examination of the consequences of the application of new technologies prior to their implementation, being mindful of the ethical issues that might be raised by these applications, and of the impacts such implementations might have on all people involved in the service-delivery system. We further commit ourselves to insisting on the widest possible discussion of the moral dilemmas that might arise, helping to articulate the choices or costs in human terms of the implementation of any technological instrument. (Palombo, 1980, pg. 311)

One specific issue, for example, is related to applications of computerized decision systems. When one consults human experts, it is recognized that they can and do make mistakes. If a decision support or expert system gives bad advice, can the designer of the system be sued? Legal issues relate to questions of ownership of programs and data, as well as the protection and the rights of all participants in the service delivery system. Concern about the confidentiality of records, however, is becoming a secondary issue since multiple safeguards are available (Mutschler, 1986). But other concerns include the danger that human services will become unresponsive to the individual's needs and values; the degree of client involvement in the evaluation and implementation of computer-assisted services; the element of control, since changed access to data might upset control or power structures in an organization; and finally, from a societal perspective, the implications of information technology on the home, the workplace, marginal groups (Nowotny, 1981), or on the way we think about ourselves (Turkle, 1984).

Computer Literacy in Human Services Education and Practice

A growing number of undergraduate and graduate human service training programs include computer support and computer instruction in their curricula. Instruction initially takes the form of demonstrations, although a growing number of institutions are acquiring sufficient resources to offer hands-on instruction in a microcomputer lab. Standard computer applications such as data base systems, statistical applications, word processing and spread sheets are the most prominent in information technology classes (Vogel, 1986).

My concern is that the aims of computer literacy for human service professionals are too often limited to proficiency in the use of the technology. However, for professionals to become leaders and architects of change, contributing to innovative uses of information technology, training and research, their training must encompass more. Human service professionals need to acquire knowledge about information and decision theory. They need to understand the functions of information within organizations. They should have the knowledge and the skills to create computer applications which will improve the delivery and outcomes of human services. Stein and Rzepnicki (1984) have identified, for example, the information practitioners need for specific intake and planning decisions in child welfare services. This information can be used to develop computerized intake and assessment procedures that allow systematic evaluation as to which procedures are most effective.

This need for sophisticated understanding and uses of technology is especially important in decision support and expert systems where uncritical acceptance of technical answers to the formulation and solution of social problems can have serious consequences; for example, faulty expert system guiding the behavior of novice practitioners. Computer literacy, in this context, reaches beyond learning to manipulate a word processor or a spread sheet. Human service professionals should possess sufficient knowledge and skills so that they, not the computer experts, can provide leadership in determining the appropriate and inappropriate uses of information technology in their respective fields.

CONCLUSION

I have described how information, decision support, and expert systems can assist the practitioner with structured, semi-and unstructured decisions in human services. Interested readers can find more detailed information in recent publications about clinical decision applications (Geiss et al., 1986; Schuerman, 1986; Schwartz, 1984), or about the development of expert systems (Hayes-Roth et al., 1984; Bennett, 1983). Much of the appeal of computerized decision applications lies in their ability to facilitate the encoding and systematic use of knowledge, rules, and facts needed for decisions that consist of a mixture of facts and subjective judgements, which are difficult to codify, yet characterize the expertise of skilled human service practitioners.

REFERENCES

Bennett, J.L. (1983). *Building Decision Support Systems*. Reading, MA: Addison Wesley.

Boyd, L., Pruger, R., Chase, M.D., Clark, M., and Miller, L.S. (1982). "A Decision Support System to Increase Equity." *Administration in Social Work*, 83-96.

Buchanan, B.G., and Shortcliffe, E.H. (1984). *Rule-Based Expert Systems: The MYCIN Experiments of the Stanford Heuristic Programming Project*. Reading, MA: Addison, Wesley.

Gambrill, E., and Stein, Th.J. (1983). *Supervision: A Decision Making Approach*. Beverly Hills: Sage Publications.

Geiss, G.R., and Viswanathan N. (Eds.) (1986). *The Human Edge*. New York: The Haworth Press, Inc.

Greist, J.H., and Klein, M.H. (1980). "Computer Programs for Patients, Clinicians, and Researchers in Psychiatry." In: J.B. Sidowski, J.H. Johnson, and T.A. Williams (Eds.) *Technology in Mental Health Care Delivery Systems.* Norwood, NJ: Ablex Publishing, 165-166.

Hayes-Roth, F., Waterman, D.A., and Lenat, D.B. (1984). *Building Expert Systems.* Reading, MA: Addison-Wesley.

Hedlund, J.L., Vieweg, B.V., and Cho, D.W. (1985). "Mental Health Computing in the 1980's: General Information Systems and Clinical Documentation." *Computers in Human Services, 1*, 3-33.

Henderson, J.C. (1986). Emerging Trends and Issues in Decision Support Systems and Related Technologies: Implications for Organizations. In: G.R. Geiss and N. Viswanathan (Eds.) *The Human Edge.* New York: The Haworth Press, Inc., 92-107.

Keen, P.G.W., and Scott-Morton, M.S. (1978). *Decision Support Systems: An Organizational Perspective.* Reading, MA: Addison-Wesley.

Lynett, P. (1986). "Information Technology in Professional Preparation and Delivery of Services. In G.R. Geiss, and N. Viswanathan (Eds.) *The Human Edge.* New York: The Haworth Press, Inc., 190-204.

Mutschler, E. (1986). "Computer Applications". In: *Encyclopedia of Social Work* (18th Edition). New York: National Association of Social Workers, 316-326.

Mutschler, E., and Hasenfeld, Y. (1985). "Integrated Information Systems for Social Work Practice." *Social Work, 31*(5), 345-349.

Nowotny, H. (1981). *The Information Society: Its Impact on the Home, Local Community and Marginal Groups.* Vienna, European Center for Social Welfare Training and Research.

Palombo, J. (1986). "The Relationship of Values to Information Technology and Clinical Social Work." In: G.R. Geiss, and N. Viswanathan (Eds.) *The Human Edge.* The Haworth Press, Inc., 305-311.

Schoech, D., Jennings, H., Schkade, L.L., and Hooper-Russell Ch. (1985). Expert Systems: Artificial Intelligence for Professional Decisions. *Computers in Human Services, 1*,(1), 81-115.

Schuerman, J.R. (1987). Expert Consulting Systems in Social Welfare. *Social Work Research and Abstracts*, in press.

Schwartz, M.D. (1984). *Using Computers in Clinical Practice: Psychotherapy and Mental Health Applications.* New York: The Haworth Press.

Scott-Morton, M. (1971). *Management Decision Systems: Computer Based Support for Decision Making.* Cambridge, MA: Division of Research, Graduate School of Business, Harvard University.

Shortcliffe, E. (1984). Reasoning Methods in Medical Consultation Systems: Artificial Intelligence Approaches. *Computer Programs in Biomedicine, 18*, 5-14.

Simon, H. (1960). *The New Science of Management Decision.* New York: Harper & Row.

Slack, W.V., and Slack, C.W. (1977). "Talking to a Computer About Emotional

Problems: A Comparative Study.'' *Psychotherapy: Theory, Research, and Practice, P, 14,* 156-164.

Turkle, Sh. (1984). *The Second Self: Computers and the Human Spirit.* New York: Simon and Schuster.

Vogel, L.H. (1986). ''Discussion of Information Technology in Professional Preparation and Delivery of Services.'' In: G.R. Geiss, and N. Viswanathan (Eds.) *The Human Edge.* New York: The Haworth Press, Inc., 205-211.

Vogel, L.H. (1985). ''Decision Support Systems in the Human Services: Discovering Limits to a Promising Technology.'' *Computers in Human Services, 1*(1), 67-80.

Developing Expert Systems

Wallace J. Gingerich

KEYWORDS. Computers, expert systems, problem selection, knowledge acquisition, knowledge representation, tools, human services, mental health.

SUMMARY. This article provides an overview of the general procedure and steps involved in developing expert systems. The first consideration is to select a suitable problem. Actual development of the expert system begins with formulating and representing the knowledge base. Then a programming tool is selected for use in developing the expert system and a working prototype is developed. After a period of evaluation and reformulation the full expert system is completed. Finally, the performance of the expert system is formally evaluated, final modifications are made, and the expert system is put into everyday use. Additional resources are provided for further reference.

If expert systems technology is to be used successfully in the human services, it must be applied selectively and competently. The first concern is selecting and formulating a problem that is suitable for expert systems technology. Often the question is not if we should develop an expert system, but rather which aspect of the problem lends itself to expert systems development.

SELECTING A SUITABLE PROBLEM

Waterman (1986) suggests that we develop an expert system only if it is possible, justified, and appropriate.

Wallace J. Gingerich is affiliated with the School of Social Welfare, University of Wisconsin-Milwaukee.

251

Is It Possible?

Genuine experts exist. Since the knowledge base of an expert system is based on that of the human expert, it is critical that a true expert be selected for the project. Human experts are generally recognized by their colleagues as experts, and they are significantly better than non-experts in solving problems in their domain of expertise. A further requirement is that the experts in an area agree among themselves on the correct solution, otherwise it will be hard to validate the expert system, or even to claim that expertise exists. At least one true expert must be available for the extensive work required to develop an expert system, and this expert must have at least minimal ability to articulate his or her method of solving the problem.

The problem is not too difficult. The problem to be transferred to the expert system must not be too hard or too easy, nor must it require a lot of common sense for its solution. The problem must be well enough understood that an expert can train someone else to do it without relying exclusively on on-the-job experience. As a general rule, the problem should be one that an expert can solve in an hour or two. If a solution takes days or weeks, the task should be broken down into subtasks which may be appropriate for expert system development. On the other hand, if the task is too easy — it can be easily learned and its solution takes only a matter of minutes — it would not be worthwhile to develop an expert system.

Only problems that require cognitive skill and specialized knowledge are suitable for expert systems. If a problem requires too much common sense knowledge it is not a good candidate because it is very difficult to transfer common sense knowledge to an expert system (Waterman, 1986), and it is possible that an expert system is not needed. On the other hand, the problem should require specialized cognitive knowledge and skill, that is, the problem should be fairly well understood and the procedures for solving it should be reasonably clear-cut and reliable.

Is It Justified?

Whether a potential application is justified depends on the nature of the expertise involved, and whether there is some benefit for the development of an expert system.

Expertise is scarce. Development of an expert system is generally justified only if human expertise is in short supply or is being lost through employee turnover or retirement. A good example of this is found in departments of social services which are responsible for investigating child abuse and neglect cases. Although staff can develop the necessary expertise over time, a study cited by Schoech et al. (1985) found that on the average child welfare staff left their positions before they developed full proficiency at some of their tasks. In such situations, an expert system would be justified because it provides scarce expertise to many professionals who need it. Once developed, it is a simple and inexpensive matter to duplicate the program and distribute it to those who need it.

Benefits are high. The benefits of developing an expert system should outweigh the costs involved. In business and industry the payoff is frequently financial, for example, one expert system, PROSPECTOR, led to the discovery of a highly valuable mineral deposit (Harmon and King, 1985). In human services the payoff is usually less tangible, for example, improved health, psychological well-being, or more satisfying relationships. Nevertheless, expert systems that identify children with learning disabilities, or children who are being abused or neglected, benefit those children significantly if the necessary services are subsequently provided. Likewise, expert systems that assist in identifying behavioral and psychological disfunction should lead to more effective intervention and thereby reduce human pain and discomfort.

Is It Appropriate?

Appropriateness has to do with the nature and scope of the problem to be addressed, and whether it lends itself to the type of problem-solving for which an expert system is capable.

Problem requires symbolic reasoning. To be appropriate for an expert system, the problem should be one that is best solved by using heuristics or rules of thumb. Further, the problem should require symbolic reasoning rather than a mathematical formula for its solution. Although this description fits most human service problems, considerable care should be given to selecting a suitable problem. If the solution can be reduced to a clear-cut formula or algorithm, then a more conventional programming approach is advised.

Scope is narrow yet practical. Problems should be sufficiently narrow in scope to be manageable, yet sufficiently broad to be useful or practical. This is one of the most difficult aspects of problem selection, partly because scope is hard to define, and partly because the tendency is to choose a problem that is too broad. For example, selecting the best reinforcer for a behavior modification program would probably be too narrow to be of much real value. On the other hand, designing an intervention program would probably be too broad, unless you are prepared to devote a great deal of time and effort to development of the expert system. A better place to start would be to develop an expert system to advise on selection of treatment strategy. Once that has been developed, a component that advises on setting up a reinforcement program, of which selecting a reinforcer may be a part, may be the next logical step.

A great deal of thought should be given to selecting the problem. Perhaps the advice of an experienced knowledge engineer (specialist in expert systems development) should be sought. The tendency will be to select too large a problem, and perhaps one that is too vague and ill-defined. Some experienced computer professionals suggest it is best to start with a problem that can be solved in about half-an-hour of consultation with a human expert. Also, it is essential that true expertise on the problem exists. If experts don't agree on the solution to the problem, then it is not suitable for expert systems development.

DEVELOPING THE EXPERT SYSTEM

Developing an expert system is a bit like doing psychotherapy. It consists of a number of stages that are overlapping and not very well defined, yet there is a general plan one follows as the process unfolds.

Knowledge Acquisition

The following discussion presumes two general roles in expert systems development, the domain expert and the knowledge engineer. The domain expert is the human expert who is recognized for her expertise in the selected problem. The domain expert's job is to be available and actively involved during the development process, particularly knowledge acquisition and testing, as directed by the knowledge engineer.

The knowledge engineer is the computer expert who knows how to develop the knowledge base and program it into the computer. The knowledge engineer's job is to direct the technical aspects of the development work such as knowledge mining, tool selection, programming and implementation. Although it may be possible for one person to be both domain expert and knowledge engineer, it is unlikely that that will lead to the best results. As the technology develops and becomes more accessible, however, it may become feasible for human service professionals to act as their own knowledge engineers in the development of small expert systems.

Select the expert. The knowledge acquisition phase begins with selecting the domain expert. Obviously, this person must be someone who has true expertise in the problem area. The expert must also be available and interested in the project. Although the time demands vary widely with the project, the domain expert will probably need to be available a minimum of a half-day a week for at least six months. Development of large systems may require participation on a half-time basis or more, over a period of months or even years. Clearly, when this level of participation is required, it is important to determine that the expert will indeed be available and willing to participate for the duration of the project. While the knowledge development process may have some interesting aspects to it, it also becomes tedious over the long term and requires substantial commitment from the domain expert.

The knowledge acquisition process. The knowledge that goes into the expert system may originate from many sources: the professional literature, practice experience, empirical studies and case studies. Thus, the knowledge engineer will usually begin by familiarizing himself with the formal knowledge of the problem as reflected in writings. But very soon, the knowledge engineer will begin interviewing the human expert in an effort to uncover or "mine" her knowledge of the problem.

The knowledge acquisition process consists mainly of an extended series of interactions between the knowledge engineer and the domain expert. These interactions usually take the form of interviews in which the knowledge engineer extracts the factual knowledge and rules of thumb the human expert uses to solve the problem. The focus must always be on how the expert solves the selected problem or task. Usually the conversation will focus on actual cases with the domain expert describing her analysis of the problem and how she went about solving it.

One technique useful in knowledge acquisition is to ask the expert to think out loud as she is solving the problem. It is often helpful to listen in on consultation sessions the expert conducts when advising on the problem. Johnson (cited in Waterman, 1986) suggests a more intuitive approach in which the domain expert introspects and builds her own theory about how she solves the problem. Sometimes it is helpful simply to watch the expert as she solves a problem. In any case, a naive but patient and painstaking approach is needed to extract the expertise of the human expert.

Knowledge acquisition is an interactive and iterative process, following what might be called a describe-analyze-refine cycle (Waterman, 1986). Often, after repeated questioning from the knowledge engineer, and solving a range of real-life problems, the domain expert will refine, revise and elaborate the facts and rules she uses. Then as the knowledge engineer translates the domain expert's knowledge into rules, the domain expert should review them. This will lead to further refinements and changes. Later, when the expert system is being evaluated, it is likely that still additional rules will need to be added and others modified. In most cases the process of knowledge development and acquisition continues indefinitely.

The process of knowledge acquisition has led to some interesting observations about the nature of expertise which may help us understand the process better. It seems to be the nature of human expertise that experts cannot readily describe how they reach their conclusions. Some have even called this the paradox of expertise (Johnson, 1983). When asked to explain their problem-solving process, experts often give general intuitive explanations which are neither very precise nor informative. Yet the problem-solving process must be described and represented specifically if the computer expert system is to perform competently. While it can be frustrating at times, this process of careful discovery and description of the problem-solving process leads to one of the important side benefits of developing an expert system, that is, our understanding of the problem-solving process will likely improve considerably.

Organizing and representing knowledge. Probably the most difficult and technical aspect of expert systems development is deciding how to represent the knowledge of the human expert in the computer system. Briefly, the three most common knowledge representation systems are rules, frames and semantic nets (Waterman, 1986). Rule-based expert systems are the most common type, and are generally the type used in diagnostic and prescriptive systems. Knowledge is represented in a series of IF-THEN rules which are checked against facts entered by the user or generated from other rules. An example of an IF-THEN rule follows.

IF: The behavior is one that is to be eliminated
AND the behavior must be eliminated fairly soon
AND the classroom and school situation is appropriate for timeout
AND characteristics of the child are appropriate for timeout,
THEN: Timeout can be recommended. (Ferrara, Serna and Baer, 1986)

Rule-based expert systems may be designed as backward-chaining, forward-chaining, or sometimes a combination. In a backward-chaining or goal-directed inference system, the system begins with the goal and looks for the first rule which might produce the goal. The system then tries to determine if the IF conditions of the rule are true. The system may query the user, or perhaps try another rule which could produce the value of the IF conditions. These IFs then become "sub-goals" and the system "backs up" to test rules as necessary until it eventually determines the value of the initial goal, hence the name backward-chaining control strategy. When the value of the goal is determined, the rule fires and the appropriate action is performed.

A forward-chaining control strategy is sometimes referred to as a data driven system. Here the system begins by looking at the rule set to find the first rule for which the IF clause is true. The rule is then fired, and the conclusion used to provide values for the IFs of other rules. As with backward-chaining systems, the parameters of the IF clauses may also be determined by asking the user for information (for example, "Is the behavior one that is to be eliminated?"). The system continues examining all the rules until no additional rules fire. The advice given is based upon the conclusions which can be inferred from the facts determined during the consultation.

The other two ways of representing knowledge, frames and semantic nets, are more complicated and are generally used in more sophisticated expert systems. Both of these methods incorporate a network type of hierarchy for representing knowledge and inferring conclusions. Some of the expert system tools are now beginning to incorporate frames, as a way to represent more complex knowledge more efficiently. Semantic nets have been used principally in natural language processing. Both frames and semantic nets are beyond the scope of this article, and are likely to be beyond the technical skill of non-computer experts to implement. The interested reader may refer to the sources listed at the end of this article for more detailed information on these methods.

Select the Programming Tool

Once the knowledge of the proposed expert system has been described and represented, it can be programmed into the computer. Small expert systems can be implemented satisfactorily on small personal computers such as the IBM PC and AT computers; larger and more sophisticated ones may require specialized and costly LISP machines.

In the area of expert systems, there are two general approaches to select from. Until recently, all expert systems were implemented in one of the artificial intelligence languages such as LISP or Prolog. Many of the more sophisticated expert systems being developed today are still implemented in programming languages because they offer the most flexibility and the best performance. Such systems, however, generally require the services of a computer programmer, and are often beyond the resources of human service agencies.

The recommended approach for most human service professionals is to use an expert system tool to implement the expert system. An expert system tool or "shell" is a computer program which has inference mechanisms, control strategies, and knowledge representation systems already built in. Such programs make development of expert systems much easier, because much of the programming is already done. While such tools do not have the flexibility and performance characteristics of a custom written expert system, they are satisfactory for many applications and they have the advantage of being accessible to non-computer professionals.

Expert systems tools have just begun to appear within the last several years. There are probably fifty or more such tools already available for personal computers, and the number is expected to increase in the next few years. Prices range anywhere from a few dollars for small "shareware" or "freeware" tools to twenty thousand dollars or more for the most sophisticated packages. As the technology matures the features of the packages will likely become more standardized, and prices will decline.

A number of considerations should be kept in mind when deciding which tool to purchase. The most important consideration is whether the tool supports the type of knowledge representation and inferencing system your problem requires. Some of the less expensive tools may be limited to a backward-chaining rule-based system, for example. Others can incorporate forward-chaining, and a few can implement frames and other more sophisticated features.

Other considerations include whether the tool is supported by the company who markets it, whether it has adequate documentation, and whether training and consultation are available if needed. Reliability and the prospect of upgrades are also important considerations. This is difficult to assess, however, because most of the companies in the current market have not been in business long enough to establish a track record, or to have their tools actually used in real life applications. Refer to the additional resources at the end of this article for up-to-date reviews of expert systems tools and languages.

Develop Prototype System

Once you have selected a tool, the next step is to do the actual programming. The immediate goal is to develop a demonstration prototype expert system which implements a small portion of the problem in order to test the design and functioning of the system. Demonstration prototypes typically include fifty to one hundred rules. They should be tested on at least a few test cases to confirm that it functions correctly. Such prototypes can usually be developed in several months.

Develop Complete System

Based on the performance of the demonstration prototype, the knowledge structure may be modified and the scope of the problem may be changed. The next step then is to proceed with full-scale development of the expert system, incorporating a complete and detailed knowledge base and well developed inference system. The complete expert system is usually refined with particular attention to its user interface, help system, and freedom from bugs. It should be a system that is relatively easy to learn and use, and one that the uninitiated user will find natural and unintimidating.

The full-scale expert system may proceed through several phases, sometimes referred to as research, field, production and commercial phases (Waterman, 1986). In actual practice, however, few expert systems have moved beyond the demonstration stage, and very few have reached the level of production or commercial systems. This no doubt reflects the considerable costs involved in development, refinement and evaluation of expert systems, and the expense involved in marketing and distribution.

Evaluate

After the full-blown system is developed it must undergo a period of testing and evaluation before being implemented in the work environment. Criteria and procedures for evaluating the performance of expert systems are still evolving (Buchanan and Shortliffe, 1984). At a minimum, however, the advice given by the expert system should be compared with that given by human experts on a subset of actual cases. The goal is for the expert system to perform at a level equal to or better than human experts. Formal evaluations have demonstrated that some systems have in fact attained this goal (Yu et al., 1984; Martindale et al., 1986).

Integrate Into Work Environment

The final stage in implementing an expert system is integrating it into the work environment. Strangely enough, some capable expert systems have not been put into day-to-day use, apparently because of insufficient planning regarding how the potential users would react to them or use them. Technology transfer is not automatic! One strategy for avoiding this problem is involving the potential users of the expert system in the initial phase of problem selection. They might also be asked to respond to the demonstration prototype, and offer suggestions. Finally, the users must be given the training necessary to use the expert system knowledgeably. If the expert system addresses a need perceived by the users, it is much more likely to be used.

This article has provided an introduction to the development of expert systems in human service practice. Expert systems technology is still relatively new, however, and its potential for supporting human service practice has yet to be demonstrated. Interested human service professionals would be well advised to consider carefully what problems might lend themselves to expert systems technology, and then evaluate these applications by developing small demonstration prototypes. As the theory and technology of expert systems develops, and the proficiency of human service professionals to use the technology increases, it is likely that genuinely useful expert systems will emerge. Hopefully, by that time some of the difficult issues related to liability and ethics will also have been resolved.

REFERENCES

Buchanan, B. G., & Shortliffe, E. H. (Eds.) (1984). *Rule-based expert systems*. Reading, MA: Addison-Wesley.

Ferrara, J. M., Serna, R. W., & Baer, R. D. (1986). *Behavior consultant: An expert system for the diagnosis of social/emotional behavioral problems* [Computer program]. Logan, UT: Utah State University, Artificial Intelligence Research and Development Unit, Developmental Center for Handicapped Persons.

Harmon, P. & King, D. (1985). *Expert systems*. New York: John Wiley & Sons.

Johnson, P. E. (1983). What kind of expert should a system be? *The Journal of Medicine and Philosophy*, 8, 77-97.

Martindale, E. S., Ferrara, J. M., & Campbell, B. W. (1986). *Accuracy of Class.LD2: An expert system for classifying learning disabled students*. Unpublished manuscript, Utah State University, Department of Special Education.

Schoech, D., Jennings, H., Schkade, L. L., & Hooper-Russell, C. (1985). Expert systems: Artificial intelligence for professional decisions. *Computers in Human Services*, 1, 81-115.

Waterman, D. A. (1986). *A guide to expert systems*. Reading, MA: Addison-Wesley.

Yu, V. L., Fagan, L. M., Bennett, S. W., Clancey, W. J., Scott, A. C., Hannigan, J. F., Blum, R. L., Buchanan, B. G., & Cohen, S. N. (1984). An evaluation of MYCIN's advice. In B. G. Buchanan and E. H. Shortliffe (Eds.), *Rule-based expert systems* (pp. 589-596). New York: Addison-Wesley.

ADDITIONAL RESOURCES

General Readings in Expert Systems

Harmon, P. & King, D. (1985). *Expert systems*. New York: John Wiley & Sons. This is probably the best introduction to the topic, especially for the uninitiated reader. It includes a description of well known systems, tools, and expert systems used for training.

Waterman, D. A. (1986). *A guide to expert systems*. Reading, MA: Addison-Wesley. More detailed and complete than Harmon and King, this is a practical guide to the development of expert systems. Includes an extensive listing of expert systems developed to date.

Hayes-Roth, F., Waterman, D. & Lenat. D. (Eds.) (1983). *Building Expert Systems*. Reading, MA: Addison-Wesley. A widely used resource on all aspects of designing and building expert systems.

Buchanan, B. G., & Shortliffe, E. H. (Eds.) (1984). *Rule-based expert systems*. Reading, MA: Addison-Wesley. Although this volume describes the work on MYCIN at Stanford University, the information it contains is applicable to expert systems in general. It is a scholarly treatment of many of the issues in knowledge representation, reasoning strategies, and implementation and evaluation.

Magazines

The AI Magazine, published by the American Association for Artificial Intelligence, 445 Burgess Drive, Menlo Park, CA 94025-3496. This is the most popular magazine on artificial intelligence for the lay reader.

AI Expert, published by CL Publications, 650 Fifth St., Suite 311, San Francisco,

CA 94107. A magazine for the general reader devoted exclusively to expert systems.

Conferences to Attend

National Conference on Artificial Intelligence. American Association for Artificial Intelligence (AAAI), 445 Burgess Drive, Menlo Park, CA 94025-3496. This is the largest single conference on the general area of AI and includes many vendor exhibits.

Symposium on Computer Applications in Medical Care. Secretariat: The George Washington University Medical Center, Office of Continuing Medical Education, 2300 K Street, N.W., Washington, D. C. 20037. This conference includes sessions and tutorials on expert systems in the medical field.

A Review of Automated Assessment

Paula S. Nurius

KEYWORDS. Assessment, mental health, clinical, testing, interviews, diagnosis, client reaction, clinical acceptance, literacy, ethics, computer supported treatment

SUMMARY. The following briefly overviews current computer tools available for clinical testing, diagnostic, and interviewing purposes. The impact of these computer-based assessment tools is then assessed in terms of empirical evidence regarding their performance and client response. The paper concludes with a discussion of training needs and issues.

The messages are ubiquitous and unmistakable. Computers are "in" — in our banking, in our shopping, in our health care, in our schools, in our homes, in our worksites, and, increasingly, in the conduct of our clinical practice. As with many technological innovations, the development and proliferation of computers initially generated an unbridled enthusiasm coupled with predictions of sweeping, revolutionary change from numerous sectors (cf., Wortman, 1981 on medical innovations). And, as the evolutionary course of innovations usually goes, consideration of the promise and pitfalls of computer technology has matured, inviting a more balanced and penetrating discourse. In keeping with this perspective, the present article encourages discussion of "second level

Paula S. Nurius, Assistant Professor at the University of Washington School of Social Work, received her doctoral training from the University of Michigan. Her current scholarship interests include the role of cognitive appraisal in stress and coping and in clinical reasoning, the self-concept, and practice evaluation as well as computer applications in direct practice.

The author would like to thank Anne Nicoll and three anonymous reviewers for their constructive comments on earlier versions of the following two papers.

questions'' regarding computer literacy and the role of computer resources in human service activities, particularly in clinical assessment.

First, current computer tools available for use in clinical testing, diagnosis, and client interviews will be briefly described. This will be followed by a review of the empirical evidence regarding the performance of and client response to these computer-based assessment tools. The article will conclude with a discussion of training needs and issues. Due to the broad scope of tools and evidence coupled with space limitations, extensive references will be provided to guide the interested reader towards detailed work on individual topics.

AN OVERVIEW OF COMPUTER-ASSISTED ASSESSMENT TOOLS

Since the development of computer technology in the 1950s, practitioners and researchers alike have been interested in discovering appropriate ways to incorporate this technology into practice. Although perceived by many to be a recent development, computers have been used as a tool in psychological assessment for more than 20 years (Fowler, 1985). Originally used principally as a means for more quickly and accurately scoring and recording personality tests scores, the capabilities of computers have been increasingly directed towards more complex uses in interviewing and diagnostic reasoning. Although a plethora of computerized tools are presently available for use by practitioners in the assessment phase of treatment, the vast majority of these have been directed toward the computer's speed, accuracy, objectivity and memory capacity; particularly speed. With respect to more flexible, creative and qualitatively different assessment strategies, we have only begun to tap the resources, and issues, that computers may offer.

Computer-Based Testing

One of the early uses of computers in practice was to take over the mundane task of scoring standardized personality tests (e.g., the MMPI, CPI, 16PF, and the Rorschach). Typically tests were administered by paper and pencil method and mailed to testing centers where large mainframe computers scored and, in some cases, provided interpretative reports on the test results. With the advent of personal computers came a major shift in convention to interactive test administration wherein it is now often the client who sits at the computer and uses the computer keyboard to indicate his/her responses to test items. As a result, the time it takes clinicians to get results from such tests has decreased from weeks to a matter of hours and, in some cases, minutes.

This translation of standardized pencil and paper tests to computerized form has been rather straightforward and has only called on some of the more basic capabilities of the computer such as displaying information on the screen, saving information entered by the client at the keyboard, and processing the algorithm used to determine a score from the data the client has provided. Because of the relative ease with which this automation process takes place, we have seen a proliferation of computerized self-report instruments generally categorized as objective tests (see Fowler, 1985 and Hedlund, Vieweg, & Cho, 1985b for extensive listings of these applications). Although to a much lesser extent, projective tests such as the Rorschach have also been computerized (Exner, 1983; Harris et al., 1981; Hopwood, Wei, & Yellin, 1981). The computerization of these types of tests will likely be enhanced by recent advances in computer graphics that allow clients to create pictures and to manipulate objects (as opposed to just text) on the screen.

Developments in computer-assisted testing have paralleled in several respects the computer literacy paradigm (see Reinoehl, this volume). Initial steps in simply automating burdensome tests to enhance efficiency reflect a beginning awareness of the computer's potential for assessment goals. A major step forward in the clinical utility of these tools was realized with development of the capacity to not only generate scores but also to generate profiles and interpretive reports. To date, the MMPI has served as something of a standard for both standardized computerized testing and interpretive programming (see, for example, Miller et al., 1977; Moreland, 1985), with increasing emphasis on producing reliable and interventionally relevant products. This step toward more interpretive functions has involved a greater degree of both technical and substantive proficiency in developing, implementing, and evaluating more complex and practice relevant capabilities. The current evidence and issues concerning these capabilities will be addressed in later sections as will emerging creative developments (e.g., tailored tests, verbal and pictoral displays; retrofit programming).

Computerized Interviewing Tools

As the realm of possibilities beyond automating standardized tests began to unfold, use of the computer in structured and interactive client interviewing began to flourish. As early as 1966, Slack, Hicks, Reid, and Van Cana reported use of a direct patient computer interview. Soon to emerge, of course, were computerized interview schedules geared to the DSM I, II, and III (Spitzer, 1983; Spitzer & Endicott, 1968, 1974). Computerized clinical interviews proliferated during the 1970s reflecting developments ranging from automating comprehensive agency intake questionnaires to sophisticated and specialized topics such as alcohol use, sexual dysfunction, and suicide risk (for review, see Erdman, Klein, & Greist, 1985 and Hedlund et al., 1985b). Recent developments have also included automation of the National Institution of Mental Health Diagnostic Interview Schedule (DIS) (Griest, Klein, Erdman, & Jefferson, 1983) and interview systems designed to facilitate evaluation of degree of client improvement in treatment over time (McCullough, 1983).

Two contrasting strategies are currently evident in the design and use of computer interviews. One approach involves broad-based interview schedules covering a wide range of areas. Examples of these include the DIS noted above, the Psychiatric Assessment Unit (Johnson, Giannetti, & Williams, 1975), and comprehensive behavioral assessments (Angle, Ellinwood, Hay, Johnsen, & Hay, 1977). These provide the obvious advantages of relieving clinicians from time-consuming, repetitive intake-type interviews while ensuring that a broad inventory of topics has been covered.

Some have questioned, however, whether this broad inventory of topics is indeed an optimal approach to interviewing. One rationale for this position, relevant to the concept of computer literacy, is that more general cognitive tasks tend to be better suited to the capabilities and strengths of the clinician whereas the more focused, repetitive (although not necessarily less complicated) tasks are better suited to the strengths of the computer (e.g., Blois, 1980). Practically speaking, the work involved with present methods of developing comprehensive interviews is often inordinate to the task — especially if many different "branches" of questions are involved or if variations in clinician style or setting requirements argue for the ability to readily tailor the program. However, as technology advances and agencies' larger management information systems become more interactive and more interventionally relevant, these issues may well diminish.

The alternative strategy is toward more specific, focused content areas. In addition to topic or population specific areas (e.g., alcohol and drug use, suicide risk, epilepsy, depression, sexual dysfunction, stuttering, marital discord), mental status examination interviews have been employed (e.g., Donnelly, Rosenberg, & Fleeson, 1970). However, in spite of the difficulties underlying use and development of comprehensive interviews, interest in those geared to facilitate psychiatric diagnosis, particularly when based on the DSM III, has been greater than interest in the specialty programs. This would suggest that, at this point in time, the relatively limited use of computer interviews, the pragmatic need for time-saving aids in standardized procedures, and the interest in improving psychiatric diagnosis serve to outweigh the arguments for more specialized computer-assisted interview tools in the minds of human service personnel.

Computerized Diagnostic Tools

Increasingly, computerized structured interviews are serving as the mechanism for making computer-generated or computer-consulted psychiatric diagnoses. An interesting duality is also evident in these design efforts. On the one hand, programs are becoming increasingly more complex, sophisticated, and "high tech." On the other hand, they are also becoming more flexible and more "user friendly" — often designed for administration by a trained lay interviewer and by clients themselves. The DIS and Spitzer's (1983) Structured Clinical Interview for DSM III are two examples. While considerable evidence has been amassed indicating that computer-generated diagnosis can be as reliable as those generated by clinicians and that clients report favorable reactions to the use of computerized tools, computer diagnosis is not yet well-established in actual practice.

It is difficult to discern the contribution of various barriers such as the up-front time and cost expenses, clinician resistance, concerns regarding reduced effectiveness with certain client groups, and so forth. Accurate diagnosis is at the very heart of clinical assessment requiring a high degree of clinical proficiency. It may be that, at this point in time, computer assistance with practice activities requiring higher levels of clinical expertise and creativity (and, likely, greater personal interest and professional investment) will encounter greater barriers to implementation relative to tasks more characterized by repetition, drudgery, and activities less central to one's professional identity. This premise has received some support in the finding that clinical consultation systems based on large banks and libraries of information have been more successful than have clinical applications having to do with clinical prediction (cf. Hedlund et al., 1980).

More recently, practitioners, particularly in the field of medicine, have attempted to develop programs that attempt to model the diagnostic expertise of an "expert" practitioner. These computer programs called expert systems or small knowledge systems attempt to codify the knowledge experts have as well as their practice wisdom that has accumulated through years of experience. These systems do not rely on conventional computer algorithms for their processing, but rather on an inference mechanism that is most commonly represented in the form of production rules. These rules are applied to the information about the client supplied by the practitioner and based on the information in the knowledge base supplied by the expert.

Although still in its infancy, the development of these systems appears promising, particularly in areas where the knowledge domain is relatively narrowly focused. For example, a system may be able to help a practitioner make diagnostic decisions in the area of child abuse or eating disorders. But, the likelihood of a system that could cover the broad knowledge domain found in the DSM III is at present not as promising. (For additional information in this area, the reader is referred to Gingerich's article in this issue.)

PERFORMANCE EVALUATIONS AND CLIENT IMPACT

As with their human and paper and pencil counterparts, computer-based assessment tools have undergone scrutiny regarding their reliability, efficacy, accuracy, and impact – both on the individual and the organization. The outcomes of these empirical evaluations have tended to be quite favorable. The computer applications that have received the most widespread acceptance and, not surprisingly, the greatest degree of controlled evaluation have been automated standardized tests and computer-based test interpretations. In reviewing and summarizing the extent to which these computer-based testing tools have achieved their goals, Fowler (1985) notes an ever increasing acceptance and user satisfaction. Also noted was the consistency of evidence to date regarding reliability and comparability to clinician administered and interpreted tests as well as a level of impact on psychological assessment that has far exceeded original expectations.

In reviews of the computer-based tests and test interpretation systems that have reported empirical evaluations, Merrell (1985), Space (1981), and Moreland (1985) found mixed although generally favorable results regarding reliability and, to a lesser degree, validity. This has been particularly true for the major personality and vocational interest inventories that have dominated the field. The current lack of instrument evaluation requirements and subsequent ease with which computer-based testing and test interpretation packages can now be developed and marketed has increased the difficulty of assessing the psychometric properties of these tools in general. Such doubts extend, of course, to any source not subject to systematic and careful evaluation – whether human or computer-based. And, as will be noted in the subsequent section, considerable debate has been generated on the validity of using clinician interpretations (as well as other aspects of assessment) as the referent for assessing the adequacy of computer-assisted assessment instruments.

With respect to computer-generated diagnoses, considerable evidence has amassed indicating these to be at least as reliable as those made by clinicians (e.g., Angle et al., 1977; Elstein, Shulman & Sprafka, 1978; Greist et al., 1983; Hedlund et al., 1980; Hedlund et al., 1985b; Mathison, Evans, Meyers, Rochford, & Wilson, 1984; Taintor, 1980). A similarly positive assessment has been rendered regarding the relative performance of computerized personal histories and interviews (e.g., Byers, 1981; Carr, Ghosh, & Ancill, 1983; Erdman et al., 1985; Helzer, Robins, Croughan, & Ratcliff, 1981; Johnson, Giannetti, & Williams, 1975, 1976; Klingler, Miller, Johnson, & Williams, 1977; Schwartz, 1984; Skinner & Allen, 1983; Slack & Slack, 1977).

More specifically, the resulting reports from systematic computer-assisted client inquiries have shown them to be more time and cost efficient, more reliable in their completeness, less susceptible to extraneous variables, and more detailed relative to traditional face-to-face methods. The advantages of greater detail and completeness have been particularly evident regarding sensitive or controversial topics wherein clients have tended to be more honest and uninhibited in their responses to computers than to human interviews (Brown, 1984; Canoune & Leyhe, 1985; Coddington & King, 1972; Evan & Miller, 1969; Hart & Goldstein, 1985; Johnson & Johnson, 1981; Lucas, Mullin, Luna, & McInroy, 1977; Merrell, 1985; Sampson, 1983; Schwartz, 1984). Examples include greater willingness to reveal sexual problems, particularly for women, and reports of significantly higher levels of alcohol consumption by individuals at alcohol treatment centers. Computerized interviews can also provide increased flexibility over paper and pencil questionnaires and inventories by being programmed to tailor questions depending on responses to previous questions (e.g., either not pursuing an irrelevant line of questioning or asking more specific questions about topics of a high individual relevance or importance).

In terms of client acceptance and reaction, the prevailing trend is that clients are generally not only not troubled by using computers for assessment purposes, but that, given a choice, a significant percentage have preferred these methods to conventional methods, including human interviewers (Klingler, Johnson, & Williams, 1976; Lucas, 1977; Maultsby & Slack, 1971; Moore, Summer, & Bloom,

1984; White, 1983). Client reports of favorable attitudes toward and experience with computer-assisted assessments have not appeared attributable to the appeal of novelty. Angle et al. (1977), for example, found this client positivity held true even for exhaustive assessments of four to ten hours. Similarly, Hart and Goldstein's (1985) electromygraph results suggest that positive attitudes and feelings toward these computerized tools does not appear attributable to demand or social desirability bias in self-reports of discomfort by clients monitored for nonvolitionally controlled stress.

Quintanor, Crowell, Pryor, and Adamopoulos (1982) recently explored the impact of various levels of "humanization" of computer usage. They found that individuals responded more positively to computer programs that appeared more human and honest. Paradoxically, however, the more human-like computers were seen by respondents as being less honest, the result being that respondents tended to be more honest and open with programs they perceived as mechanistic. In short, client reaction has generally been consistently and somewhat surprisingly positive. As the general population, particularly the youth, are becoming increasingly computer savvy, concern with client reaction may tend to fade. This would be premature. As with any component of treatment we need to know not just "does it work," but what types of clients or client problems/circumstances are these computer aids most and least successful with and why.

An area that has as yet not been well investigated involves response differences based on anxiety or unfamiliarity with the computer. Unfamiliarity with computers is likely to be more evident among women, ethnic minorities, and the aged, disabled, and poor—the very persons most likely to be seen in human service agencies. There is some tentative evidence suggesting that initial anxiety caused by the computer is short-lived when given adequate practice (Lushene, O'Neil, & Dunn, 1974; Johnson & White, 1980) and that, in some cases, responses may be facilitated through computer programmed strategies (Griest & Klein, 1980; Johnson & Mihal, 1973). Yet clear societal inequities exist regarding accessibility to and familiarity with computer technology, and concerns regarding potential jeopardy to assessment outcomes are warranted. It has been noted that computer illiteracy may be an attribute shared by all disadvantaged groups in the new era of sophisticated information technology (Geiss, 1983). The potential for discouragement and discrimination must be vigilantly monitored.

One promising trend is that computers have been successfully used with and received by client groups for whom some may have presumed its use was contraindicated. Examples of such client groups have included acute psychiatric patients (Bailine, Katzoff, & Rau, 1977; Mathison et al., 1984), individuals at risk for suicide (Greist et al., 1973), and clients with profound handicaps (Glenn, 1983), and developmental disabilities (Gardner & Brewer, 1985). Again, the research to date is neither extensive nor well-orchestrated. Clinicians must be aware of potential sources of disadvantage and work to remove or compensate for these. Fortunately, current developmental efforts appear to be attentive to some of these barriers and are experimenting with various media and methods of normalizing and facilitating use of the computer.

CONCLUSION

In addressing the present-day skills and knowledge needed to be computer literate in practice-relevant technology, it is not clear what computer abilities *per se* should be prioritized. Schools of social work, for example, are struggling with questions of how curriculum content allocations should be made among conceptual understanding, attitudes and comfort, hands-on skills, programming ability, creative thinking, and analysis of unprecedented issues and consequences. On the one hand, we hear that acute deficits in adequate training or resources for training in addition to bewildering changes associated with rapid technological advances often result in high levels of frustration, conflict, and, at times, abandonment of computerization ventures (e.g., Young, 1984). On the other hand, the late 1970s and early 1980s have produced ever-increasingly user-friendly software (such as sophisticated database management systems, interview drivers, branching test construction programs, and report writers) that require very little technical know-how for development and even less for use of the resultant applications (see Hedlund et al., 1985a and Hudson et al., 1987, for examples). Increasingly, software packages are interactive and equipped with self-contained menus and documentation that lead the user through a series of questions and prompts.

The amount and type of computer ability needed to be computer literate in automated assessment depends not surprisingly, on the type of tool used. At present there is a broad spectrum from complex and comprehensive standardized testing and diagnostic systems on mainframe computers to the very focused and simple testing devices designed for use by nonliterate clients. There does appear to be general agreement that, at a minimum, conceptual understanding of the mechanisms, strengths and limitations of the automated tool is needed. In addition, comfort with and compatible attitudes regarding the computer as a clinical aid appear important aspects of becoming computer literate.

Interestingly, "hands-on" technical training is generally not deemed as important by human service agency administrators as conceptual training and does not appear significantly correlated with new practitioners' willingness to seek future computer training. It has, however, been found to be significantly correlated with these practitioners' perceptions of their current knowledge of computers and their confidence in future mastery of computer skills. Moreover, these correlations have been found significantly higher for hands-on relative to more didactic training (Nurius, Richey, & Nicoll, 1988; Nurius, Hooyman, & Nicoll, 1987).

There also appears converging agreement of the increasing role of computers in practice activities such as assessment, and of the need for practitioners to be informed participants in design as well as usage (e.g., Schoech, 1985). What is less clear is what, during this period of technological transition, constitutes optimal training and preparation for meaningful computer literacy.

The above suggests that there is presently neither a definitive nor a universal answer regarding what should be taught to practitioners who will be using computerized assessments in practice. However, to establish a functional level of proficiency, the following are generally needed: understanding of basic computer operations and concepts; hands-on experience to enhance familiarity, comfort, and confidence; a balanced, open attitude regarding use of computers in direct service functions such as assessment; and a conceptual understanding of the substantive task at hand.

Two additional factors are important, and these begin to truly distinguish different levels of literacy. One of these is the ability to operationalize one's assessment questions, interests, or tasks in terms of the available hardware and software resources. This is particularly true when the automated assessment tools involve more than computerized analogues of conventional paper and pencil tests.

The second factor is the ability to conceptualize what the hardware and software resources *could* provide or affect (both positively and negatively). That is, the ability to creatively problem-solve, to envision possibilities, and to think in synthesized terms of the assessment aims and the technology. These latter factors will only come with experience, but training that emphasizes how to creatively and critically *think about* computer applications in addition to the more reassuring yet less generalizable "what to do's" are increasingly becoming of prime importance.

The present review of contemporary computer-based client assessment tools has drawn almost exclusively from the published professional literature. This information resource is, of course, one of the most widely accessible, professionally monitored, and traditionally used. However, with advancement of computer technology has come an additional set of information resources — specifically, various libraries, bulletin boards, and information networks accessible via telecommunication. One example of particular relevance to the present article is CUSSnet. CUSSnet is a subnetwork of a larger international electronic network (FIDONET). In addition to supporting local bulletin boards and national and local mail and file transfers, CUSSnet permits downloading of public domain software and access to repositories of electronically available information germane to human services (CUSS Network, 1986).

This alternative set of resources is noted with caution. On the one hand, applications and software relevant to direct service activities are among the most rapidly growing within the human service realm. Not infrequently, packages will be developed, implemented, and available to others long before they will appear, if ever, in the published professional literature. Many times, the interest of the developer is primarily that of meeting his/her service or practice needs and simply making these products available to others.

The caution is that such tools will frequently be available without benefit of systematic empirical validation or impact evaluation. Additional questions, several of which are addressed in the next paper, will not yet have been adequately dealt with to ensure appropriate usage of the tool. However, the role of these electronic media in making innovative practice tools rapidly and widely available will undoubtedly become increasingly normative. It will be the responsibility of the practice community to proactively develop standards and norms regarding appropriate and ethical use of emerging tools, and to participate on an informed basis in shaping future directions.

REFERENCES

Angle, H. W., Ellinwood, E. H., Hay, W. M., Johnsen, T., & Hay, L. R. (1977). Computer-aided interviewing in comprehensive behavioral assessment. *Behavior Therapy, 8,* 747-754.

Bailine, S., Katzoff, A., & Rau, J. H. (1977). Diagnosis of schizophrenia by computer and clinicians: A pilot study. *Comprehensive Psychiatry, 18*(2), 141-145.

Blois, M. S. (1980). Clinical judgment and computers. *New England Journal of Medicine, 303,* 192-197.

Brown, D. T. (1984). Automated assessment systems in school and clinical psychology: Present status and future directions. *School Psychology Review, 13*(14), 455-460.

Byers, A. P. (1981). Psychological evaluation by means of an on-line computer. *Behavior Research Methods and Instrumentation, 13*(4), 585-587.

Canoune, H. L. & Leyhe, E. W. (1985). Human versus computer interviewing. *Journal of Personality Assessment, 49*(1), 103-106.

Carr, A. C., Ghosh, A., & Ancill, R. J. (1983). Can a computer take a psychiatric history? In M. Shepherd (Ed.), *Psychological medicine*. Cambridge: Cambridge Press.

Coddington, R. D. & King, T. L. (1972). Automated history taking in child psychology. *American Journal of Psychiatry, 129,* 276-282.

CUSS Network (1986). Networking: The linking of people, resources and ideas. *Computer Use in Social Services Network, 6*(2).

Donnelly, J., Rosenberg, M., & Fleeson, W. P. (1970). The evolution of the mental status—past and future. *American Journal of Psychiatry, 126,* 997-1002.

Elstein, A. S., Shulman, L. S., & Sprafka, S. A. (1978). *Medical problem solving: An analysis of clinical reasoning*. Cambridge, MA: Harvard University Press.

Erdman, H. P., Klein, M. H., & Greist, J. H. (1985). Direct patient computer interviewing. *Journal of Consulting and Clinical Psychology, 53*(6), 760-773.

Evan, W. M. & Miller, J. R. (1969). Differential effects on response bias of computer vs. conventional administration of a social science questionnaire: An exploratory methodological experiment. *Behavioral Sciences, 14*, 216-227.

Exner, J. (1985). *The Exner report for the Rorschach comprehensive system.* Minneapolis, MN: National Computer System.

Fowler, R. D. (1985). Landmarks in computer-assisted psychological assessment. *Journal of Consulting and Clinical Psychology, 53*(6), 748-759.

Gardner, J. M. & Breuer, A. (1985). Reliability and validity of a microcomputer assessment system for developmentally disabled persons. *Education and Training of the Mentally Retarded, 20*(3), 209-213.

Geiss, G. (1983). Some thoughts about the future: Information technology and social work practice. *Practice Digest, 6*(3), 33-35.

Glenn, S. M. (1983). The application of an automated system for the assessment of profoundly handicapped children. *International Journal of Rehabilitation Research, 6*(3), 358-360.

Greist, J. H., Jefferson, J. W., Combs, A. M., Schou, M., & Thomas, A. (1977). The Lithium Librarion: An international index. *Archives of General Psychiatry, 134*, 456-459.

Greist, J. H., & Klein, M. H. (1980). Computer programs for patients, clinicians, and researchers in psychiatry. In J B. Sidowski, J. H., Johnson, & T. A. Williams (Eds.), *Technology in mental health care delivery systems* (pp. 161-182). Norwood, NJ: Ablex.

Greist, J. H., Klein, M. H., Erdman, H. P., & Jefferson, J. W. (1983). Computers and psychiatric diagnosis. *Psychiatric Annals, 13*(10), 785, 789-792.

Harris, W. G., Niedner, D., Feldman, C., Fink, A., & Johnson, J. H. (1981). An on-line interpretive Rorschach approach: Using Exner's comprehensive system. *Behavior Research Methods and Instrumentation, 13*(4), 588-591.

Hart, R. R. & Goldstein, M. A. (1985). Computer-assisted psychological assessment. *Computers in Human Services, 1*(3), 69-75.

Hedlund, J. L., Evenson, R. C., Sletten, I. W., & Cho, D. W. (1980). The computer and clinical prediction. In J. B. Sidowski, J. H. Johnson, & T. A. Williams (Eds.), *Technology in mental health care delivery systems.* Norwood, NJ: Ablex.

Hedlund, J. L., Vieweg, B. W., & Cho, D. W. (1985a). Mental health computing in the 1980s: I. General information systems and clinical documentation. *Computers in Human Servcies, 1*(1), 3-33.

Hedlund, J. L., Vieweg, B. W., & Cho, D. W. (1985b). Mental health computing in the 1980's: II. Clinical applications. *Computers in Human Services, 1*(2), 1-31.

Helzer, J. D., Robins, L. N., Croughan, J. L., & Ratcliff, K. S. (1981). National Institute of Mental Health Diagnostic Interview Schedule: Its history, characteristics and validities. *Archives of General Psychiatry, 38*, 381-389.

Hopwood, J. H., Wei, K. H., & Yellin, A. M. (1981). A computerized method for generating the Rorschach's structural summary from the sequence of scores. *Journal of Personality Assessment, 45*(2), 116-117.

Hudson, W. W., Nurius, P. S., & Reisman, S. (1987). Computerized assessment instruments: Their promise and problems. *Computers in Human Services*, in press.

Johnson, D. F. & Mihal, W. L. (1973). Performance of blacks and whites in computerized versus manual testing environments. *American Psychologist*, *28*, 694-699.

Johnson, D. F. & White, C. B. (1980). Effects of training on computerized test performance in the elderly. *Journal of Applied Psychology*, *65*, 357-358.

Johnson, J. H., Giannetti, R. A., & Williams, T. A. (1975). Real-time psychological assessment and evaluation of psychiatric patients. *Behavior Research Methods and Instrumentation*, *7*, 199-200.

Johnson, J. H., Giannetti, R. A., & Williams, T. A. (1976). Computers in mental health care delivery: A review of the evolution toward interventionally relevant on-line processing. *Behavior Research Methods and Instrumentation*, *8*(2), 83-91.

Johnson, J. H. & Johnson, K. N. (1981). Psychological considerations related to the development of computerized testing stations. *Behavior Research Methods and Instrumentation*, *13*(4), 421-424.

Klingler, D. E., Johnson, J. H., & Williams, T. A. (1976). Strategies in the evolution of an on-line computer-assisted unit for intake assessment of mental health patients. *Behavior Research Methods and Instrumentation*, *8*, 95-100.

Klingler, D. E., Miller, D. A., Johnson, J. H., & Williams, T. A. (1977). Process evaluation of an on-line computer-assisted unit for intake assessment of mental health patients. *Behavior Research Methods and Instrumentation*, *9*(2), 110-116.

Lucas, R. W. (1977). A study of patients' attitudes to computer interrogation. *International Journal of Man-Machine Studies*, *9*, 69-86.

Lucas, R. W., Mullin, P. J., Luna, C. B. X., & McInroy, D. C. (1977). Psychiatrists and a computer as interrogators of patients with alcohol-related illnesses: A comparison. *British Journal of Psychiatry*, *131*, 160-167.

Lushene, R. B., O'Neil, H. F., & Dunn, T. (1974). Equivalent validity of a computerized MMPI. *Journal of Personality Assessment*, *38*, 353-361.

Mathison, K. S., Evans, F. J., Meyers, K., Rochford, J. M., & Wilson, G. (1984, January). *An evaluation of computerized DSM-III diagnosis in a private psychiatric hospital*. Paper presented at the 51st Annual Meeting of the National Association of Private Psychiatric Hospitals, Palm Springs, CA.

Maultsby, M. O. & Slack, W. V. (1971). A computer-based psychiatry history system. *Archives of General Psychiatry*, *25*, 570-572.

McCullough, L. (1983). The development of a microcomputer based information system for psychotherapy research. *Problem Oriented Systems and Treatment Post*, *6*(1), 3-4.

Merrell, K. W. (1985). Computer use in psychometric assessment: Evaluating benefits and potential problems. *Computers in Human Services*, *1*(3), 59-67.

Miller, D. A., Johnson, J. H., Klingler, D. E., Williams, T. A., & Giannetti, R.

A. (1977). Design for an on-line computerized system for MMPI interpretation. *Behavior Research Methods and Instrumentation, 9*(2), 117-122.

Moore, N. C., Summer, K. R., & Bloor, R. N. (1984). Do patients like psychometric testing by computer? *Journal of Clinical Psychology, 40*(3), 875-877.

Moreland, K. L. (1985). Validation of computer-based test interpretations: Problems and prospects. *Journal of Consulting and Clinical Psychology, 53*(6), 816-825.

Nurius, P. S., Hooyman, N., & Nicoll, A. E. (1987). *A survey of current and future computer utilization in social work settings.* Paper presented at the Council on Social Work Education Annual Program Meeting, March, St. Louis, Missouri.

Nurius, P. S., Richey, C. A., & Nicoll, A. E. (1988). Preparation for computer usage in social work: Student consumer variables. *Journal of Social Work Education*, in press.

Quintanar, L. R., Crowell, C. R., Pryor, J. B., & Adamopoulos, J. (1982). Human-computer interaction: A preliminary social psychological analysis. *Behavior Research Methods and Instrumentation, 14*, 210-220.

Sampson, J. P. (1983). Computer-assisted testing and assessment: Current status and implications for the future. *Measurement and Evaluation in Guidance, 15*(3), 293-299.

Schoech, D. (1985). A microcomputer-based human service information system. In S. Slavin (Ed.), *Managing finances, personnel, and information in human services, vol. II of Social administration – The management of social services* (2nd ed.). New York: Haworth Press.

Schwartz, M. D. (1984). Reviews of assessment of psychiatric patients' problems by computer interview. In M. D. Schwartz (Ed.), *Using computers in clinical practice*. New York: Haworth Press.

Skinner, H. A. & Allen, B. A. (1983). Does the computer make a difference? Computerized versus face-to-face versus self-report assessment of alcohol, drug, and tobacco use. *Journal of Consulting and Clinical Psychology, 51*(2), 267-275.

Slack, W. V., Hicks, G. P., Reed, C. Z., & Van Cura, L. J. (1966). A computer-based medical history system. *New England Journal of Medicine, 274*, 194-198.

Slack, W. V. & Slack, C. W. (1977). Talking to a computer about emotional problems: A comparative study. *Psychotherapy: Theory, Research and Practice, 14*(2), 156-164.

Space, L. G. (1981). The computer as psychometrician. *Behavior Research Methods and Instrumentation, 13*(4), 595-606.

Spitzer, R. L. (1983). Are clinicians still necessary? *Comprehensive Psychiatry, 24*(5), 400-411.

Spitzer, R. L. & Endicott, J. (1968). DIAGNO: A computer program for psychiatric diagnosis utilizing the differential diagnostic procedure. *Archives of General Psychiatry, 18*, 746-756.

Spitzer, R. L. & Endicott, J. (1974). Can the computer assist clinicians in psychiatric diagnosis? *American Journal of Psychiatry, 131*(5), 523-530.

Taintor, Z. C. (1980). Computers and diagnosis [Editorial]. *American Journal of Psychiatry, 137*(1), 61-63.

White, D. M. (1983). *An assessment of the comparability of a computer administration and standard administration of the MMPI.* Unpublished master's thesis, University of Alabama.

Wortman, P. M. (1981). Randomized clinical trials. In P. M. Wortman (Ed.), *Methods for evaluating health services.* Beverly Hills, CA: Sage.

Young, T. R. (1984, April 10). The lonely micro. *Datamation 100*, 102-103, 106.

Computer Literacy
in Automated Assessment:
Challenges and Future Directions

Paula S. Nurius

KEYWORDS. Assessment, mental health, clinical, testing, interviews, diagnosis, client reaction, clinical acceptance, literacy, ethics, computer supported treatment

SUMMARY. The following paper addresses significant questions and challenges to defining and pursuing computer literacy in the realm of assessment. This includes attention to practitioner concerns as well as validity and ethical issues. The paper concludes with discussion of promising future directions, including capitalizing on the unique characteristics of the computer and qualitatively different assessment paradigms. A balanced recognition of both the promise and the potential pitfalls of computer-assisted assessment is advocated here, as well as initiative by practitioners to assume leadership roles in shaping the synthesis of computers and clinical practice.

As with most innovations, along with the promise and advantages offered by computer technology in clinical assessment have come a host of challenges and knotty issues, some without precedence. It is beyond the scope of this paper to attempt to deal with these comprehensively. Instead, the focus will be on topics germane to the formulation and pursuit of computer literacy in human services. With respect to significant challenges, the topics that will

---

Paula S. Nurius, Assistant Professor at the University of Washington School of Social Work, received her doctoral training from the University of Michigan. Her current scholarship interests include the role of cognitive appraisal in stress and coping and in clinical reasoning, the self-concept, and practice evaluation as well as computer applications in direct practice.

be addressed here include practitioner reactions, validation dilemmas and ethical issues. This will be followed by distinctions between simply automating "old" tests and designing "new" tests better suited to capitalize on the unique features of the computer. The article will conclude with discussion of promising future directions including the computer's influence in opening up qualitatively different assessment paradigms.

CHALLENGES TO DEFINING AND PURSUING COMPUTER LITERACY

Practitioner Reactions

In marked contrast to client reactions, clinicians have reacted to the use of these tools with greater hesitancy. Fowler (1985) reviewed the history and development of computer-assisted psychological assessment and surmised that fear of and negativism toward computing is "a malady that afflicts professionals much more than their patients" (p. 754). Clinicians, unfamiliar with computer applications often assert their clients would feel dehumanized and would never agree to take a test or interview on a computer, whereas experience indicates clients are seldom reluctant to do so. Johnson and Williams (1980), for example, found client response to be strongly favorable to computer testing, whereas staff attitudes ranged from neutral to somewhat negative. Carr and Ghosh (1983) found that even phobic clients indicated no apprehension about completing an assessment on the computer.

In exploring the reasons for widespread negativism and "resistance" on the part of practitioners, Hedlund, Vieweg, and Cho (1985) point to the frustration and irritation many practitioners have experienced with computer applications, various types of broad-based management information systems in particular. While clinicians have traditionally borne the input burden, they have not encountered significant benefits and have more typically experienced this task as an intrusion and barrier to clinical pursuits (see also Conklin, 1981 and Hammer & Hile, 1985). These prior experiences coupled with fears of being replaced by computers as well as some very legitimate questions about risk and compromises have negatively influenced attitudes and feelings about the potential utility of the computer in more direct clinical functions. This negativism, however, is neither uniform nor intractable. Klonoff and Clark (1975), for example, found level of knowledge and degree of involvement to be the two variables most associated with attitudes about computer applications, and that these significantly improved over a two-and-a-half-day course on computers. These findings suggest that barriers are attributable in part to the failure of clinicians to recognize the potential relevance and utility of computer applications, and to the failure of computer specialists and administrators to reckon with and draw upon the needs and expertise of the actual user—the direct practitioner.

Hammer and Hile (1985) have identified two sets of factors that appear to influence clinicians' resistance to automation in mental health: structural variables (e.g., cognitive style, perceived client resistance, questions of efficacy, value conflicts, goals conflicts, power and status issues, and legal and ethical concerns) and process variables (e.g., time and effort expenditures, problems with poor documentation and inadequate training, organizational change issues). The reasons for controversies and resistance are complex, varied, and multileveled. These perceived barriers are natural and inherent elements of the process of adapting new technology to the purposes of the agency and the profession, and by no means should be categorically viewed as inappropriate or irrational. On the contrary, several legitimate and important points have been raised and serve as useful checks on potentially unbridled enthusiasm for and embracement of these organizational and technological advances (see Hoshino, 1981; Geiss, 1983).

Staff attitudes are also important with respect to the validity and reliability of computer-assisted assessment. Lack of standardization in the administration of these tests and interviews or confounding messages, implicit or explicit, to the client could easily negatively influence an otherwise reliable and valid instrument or program. Increasingly, it is becoming clear that treating the introduction of computers solely as a technological innovation is not sufficient (e.g., Byrnes & Johnson, 1981; Drazen & Seidel, 1984; Gelernter & Gelernter, 1984; Hammer & Hile, 1985; Johnson et al., 1978). Education, involvement and considerable preparation for organizational change are needed. The reduction of threat and uncertainty is central to the successful introduction of any new technology (Baer, Johnson, & Merrow, 1977), and particularly so with a technology that has limited precedence and is constantly changing. As clinicians gain greater computer literacy vis-à-vis their human service requirements, abilities and potentialities, their attitudes are also likely to change. Yet the issues simply cannot be dismissed as clinician "techno-fright." A central future task will be to design systems better tailored to practice realities with more favorable burden-to-benefit ratios and with greater input from and relevance to line staff at each stage of development, implementation and ongoing system evaluation (e.g., Craig, 1984; Johnson, William, Klingler, & Giannetti, 1977).

Validation Dilemmas and Ethical Issues

To acquire evidence on the validity of any instrument, one or more external criteria are necessary against which to meaningfully and reliably compare the performance or outcome of the instrument in question. With such phenomena as computer-generated test interpretations and diagnoses, questions of reliability can be relatively easily investigated with repeated administrations across testers, time, circumstances, and so forth. Assessing validity, however, is much more difficult, requiring comparative standards or referents of sound performance and conceptual integrity. One obvious referent is clinician-based interpretations and diagnosis. Yet one of the major impetuses for developing descriptive rule-driven test interpretations and structured interviews for assessing psychopathology is the lack of faith or clear evidence regarding validity of clinician-generated diagnoses and interpretations. For example, a recent report of validity testing of the DIS, the NIMH diagnostic interview (Robins, Helzer, Ratcliff et al., 1982) concluded that typical clinical practice is not an adequate standard against which to assess the validity of alternative instruments. Part of the basis for this conclusion was an information deficiency—such as the frequent lack of sufficient symptoms to meet DSM III, the lack of secondary diagnoses and related missing data in client files (see also Carr, Ghosh, & Ancill, 1983; Skinner & Allen, 1983). This conclusion has also been ventured by others noting the frequent lack of agreement among clinicians as to definitions, diagnoses and interpretations as well as various forms of clinician bias (e.g., Graham & Lily, 1984; Greist, Klein, & Erdman, 1976; McDermott, 1980; Spitzer, 1983).

Questions regarding the equivalency of computer and clinician-based assessment strategies have also focused on the distinguishing features and shortcomings of the computer. For example, studies indicating higher levels of client acceptance and self-disclosure with computer-administered assessments should suggest caution rather than assumptions of the superiority of computerized methods. Such findings indicate both quantitative and qualitative differences in content provided by the client as well as "relational" differences that do not support presumptions of interchangeable equivalence between computerized and noncomputerized strategies, even of the same assessment instrument. Computerized assessment strategies raise unprecedented questions of totally new forms of "bias" — particularly computer response set bias by clients (see Hofer & Green [1985] for a review of various forms of response set bias and the implications these hold for equivalence).

Concerns about the biasing (and potentially invalidating) effects of response sets are not new (cf. Block, 1965) and are in need of further study. Duthie (1984), for example, has questioned whether the gains in time efficiency are not seriously offset by reduced client reflection on the questions posed to them and on their responses using interactive, computerized methods. Johnson and Johnson (1981) speak to the need for better understanding of how humans go about interacting with today's computers to reduce error as well as unplanned response set bias. This issue becomes even more important as new assessment strategies, such as those based on adaptive testing, that are designed specifically to suit the characteristics and capabilities of the computer.

The issues raised above and elsewhere in the paper underscore the importance of informed practice and administrative judgment in utilizing computer assessment tools in an ethically and clinically sound manner. To render sound judgments will require at a minimum an awareness of the capabilities of the computerized tool — its strengths, limitations, and unknowns. More realistically, a more in-depth understanding of the tool's capabilities and appropriateness *vis-à-vis* the practice needs and constraints of the client, problem, clinician, or intervention in question is needed. In short, current and future decisions will need to be based not on whether one is on or off the "computer bandwagon." Rather, each decision will require thoughtful and balanced consideration of the technological and practice trade-offs. For a compendium of writings addressing these and related issues relevant to human services, see the edited collection of Geiss and Viswanathan (1986).

These and related questions regarding standards are beginning to be addressed with rapidly increasing frequency within the professional literature and among policymakers. Guidelines are presently being drafted by a host of professional groups as well as computerized test publishers and distributors (see Hofer & Green, 1985, pp. 827-828 for details). Issues of ethics and sound use of computers in practice constitute a broad and complex set of topics. The interested reader is referred to the following for in-depth treatment of these topics (Buros, 1978; Hofer & Green, 1985; Johnson, 1984; Levitan, Willis, & Vogelgesang, 1985; Matarazzo, 1983; Sampson & Pyle, 1983; Turkington, 1984; Zachary & Pope, 1984). The primary goal in the present paper is to stress that the knottiest questions of computers in practice are those requiring a thorough understanding of both the technological features of the computer and the organizational and substantive realities of practice in human service settings. Our training programs for emerging practitioners must, therefore, strive to promote this more integrative and creative approach to practice-relevant computer literacy.

The above concern with training touches upon a final consideration regarding valid and ethical use of computer-based assessment tools. This has to do with issues of professional preparation and sanction. Very real and serious concerns have been raised regarding the access of computer-based assessment tools to those who are neither adequately trained to use them nor sufficiently accountable to standards of confidentiality, legitimacy and avoidance of economic and legal abuses. Should traditional lines of professional "turf" be used as guides in developing credentialing standards (e.g., personality and clinical psychologists in testing, psychiatrists in psychiatric diagnosis) for sanctioning utilization of computer applications? What of social workers and other allied helping professionals? Given (1) that evidence to date questions the equivalence of computerized and noncomputerized assessment instruments and (2) that qualitatively new and distinct computer assessment innovations are now and will continue to emerge, are former rationales and referents for establishing standards and domains of professional influence adequate to meet the changing need? These and related questions suggest the need to press the notion of computer literacy as it applies to direct practice with clients beyond its usefulness as a conceptual paradigm. It is a question of policy—actually, a complex set of policy issues—and one that is incumbent upon all human service professionals to respond to thoughtfully, thoroughly and openly. The question is no longer whether, but rather how and by whom will the roles of computers in clinical practice be determined and shaped.

COMPUTERIZING "OLD" VERSUS "NEW" TESTS

As noted, efforts to evaluate the utility of the computer for assessment purposes and the validity and reliability of instruments and products used to do so have been complicated by questions of what to use as the referent or standard against which to compare performance. Additionally, questions are raised concerning the most appropriate types of applications. What, for example, is really being tested in evaluations primarily centered around (1) conventional assessment methods that have simply been automated as compared to (2) applications developed specifically for the features of the computer that are unique and that distinguish it from conventional methods? Simply mimicking in automated form what has been done before in nonautomated ways does not take advantage of the computer's special strengths and potential (Giannetti & Klingler, 1980; Hedlund et al., 1985; Johnson, 1979; Space, 1981). Herein lies one of the greatest challenges and prospects in the future of computer-assisted practice. Moreover, it speaks to the need for greater use of a computer literacy formulation in developing these tools; of creatively blending the unique attributes of computer technology with the expertise and activities of greatest interventional relevance.

Innovations are increasingly being developed. The use of computers in interactive videos and in picture-preference versus verbal items is currently underway (Morf, Alexander, & Fuerth, 1981; Schwartz, 1981, 1984). This development is of particular importance in reducing access and usage barriers to computer technology for clients who are unable to read (e.g., young children, developmentally disabled, illiterate individuals, nonnative speakers). In addition, use of computers to record ancillary data such as response latencies and pressure on response keys has proven to be highly reliable and significantly related to a number of practice-relevant behavior patterns (Stout, 1983). The collection of physiological and neurological data are well-suited to computers and have wide applications possibilities (Beresford, Law, Hall, Adduci, & Goggans, 1982; Ropper, Griswold, McKenna, & Saunder, 1981; Space, 1981). Clinical consultation systems drawing on large bibliographic data bases have also proven successful (e.g., Erdman, 1983; Greist, Jefferson, Combs, Schou, & Thomas, 1977). Finally, the ease with which computers can now be programmed makes possible their use in providing streamlined test procedures (Butcher, Keller, & Bacon, 1985; Johnson 1979; Weiss, 1985) that ask specific items relevant to a particular client or situation and refrain from presenting questions determined to be irrelevant to a particular client on the basis of responses to prior questions.

The question of what to use as evaluative norms in comparing computerized "old" tests and interviews to conventional administration is paralleled by investigation of "new" technology for which conventional counterparts are not available (see Brown, 1984 and Moreland, 1985 for further discussion). In several respects, the rapid increase in technological advances in the hardware and software supporting assessment and practice applications have far outstripped our capacity to use, much less validate, their performance and potential. As Greist (1984) put it,

> We do not need another generation of computers or even of programming languages. We need a generation of clinicians who will take the powerful tools presently available and apply them with care, ingenuity, diligence, and patience to difficult mental health problems, which will gradually yield to our steady efforts. (p. 194)

CONCLUSIONS AND FUTURE DIRECTIONS

At this point in time, both the problems and the promises of computer-assisted assessment are significant. By and large, the view that the sound advantages outweigh the sound criticisms, and that the computer offers a unique complimentary (rather than supplanting) role is a representative and well-supported perspective. One of the most pressing areas of need is more systematic and thorough evaluation of computerized tools. Of the work done thus far, the focus has been on reliability, conceptualizing computer-assisted and conventional methods as alternate forms of the same instrument, and on convergent validity, conceptualizing the two methods as separate and distinct instruments. As noted earlier, much more extensive and refined validation research is called for as is creative research focused on more fully utilizing the computer's capacities, and on the relation of the computer to other aspects of clients' and the practitioners' thoughts, feelings, and actions.

Toward this goal, several writers have offered suggestions for future validation efforts. Farrell (1984), for example, outlines general guidelines for determining when computerized assessment systems are ready for distribution. Farrell speaks to criteria related to the computer aspect of computerized assessment systems as well as the assessment aspect of these systems. In addition to adherence to well-established principles of test construction, the importance of several forms of reliability (e.g., consistency of scores over time, internal consistency, interrater/interjudge reliability, equivalency of scores obtained from computerized and conventional versions) and of validity (e.g., content, construct, predictive, procedural) are stressed. The need for standards, for accountability, and for incentives to take on the painstaking task of evaluation in the face of pressures to move newly developed systems quickly to market are greatly needed. For discussion of needed characteristics of future validation studies, see Harris (1984), Hofer and Bersoff (1983), and Moreland (1985).

Greist et al. (1973) have pointed out a troublesome tradeoff. That is, greater specificity and systematic coverage tends to increase the reliability and validity of assessment systems yet it also tends to make their use more difficult (e.g., tedious, boring, time consuming). This is part of the impetus to move to interactive systems and to provide immediate (or close to) feedback to the user. The capability for continuous updating of the case *and* of the system has also been argued as a requirement to enhance sensitivity and utility as well as reliability and validity. Additionally, emphasis has been placed on keeping computer-generated reports brief, focused, concise, and including interventionally-relevant information (Brooks & Kleinmentz, 1974; Johnson et al., 1976; Miller et al., 1977).

The evolution of computer applications in psychological assessment has reached a stage of exciting and unprecedented potential. Whereas many of the applications to date have been of a derivative nature, we are now entering an era of far more creative and truly innovative possibilities. As previously noted, more dynamic formats for presenting stimuli and eliciting responses are beginning to be developed and tested. These include, among others: use of free response versus forced choice formats, of pictoral displays and interactive video disks and games, of speech analyzers and physiological monitoring devices, of measuring reaction times and key pressure as a basis for inferences about underlying cognitive processes, and of systematically analyzing patterns of item responses through configural scoring, factor or cluster analyses, and related analytical procedures.

Another major breakthrough has been the expansion from rigid, linear presentational models to more flexible, tailored "adaptive" testing paradigms. Adaptive tests present different sets of test questions (drawing from a much larger preprogrammed pool) depending on the nature of the respondent's answers to prior questions posed. In this fashion, each test is individually shaped by selecting items from the pool so that the characteristics of the items are adapted and thus appropriate to the characteristics of the respondent during the process of testing. Along with the advantages of greater efficiency and precision have come unique computational comparison problems. Their potential—both technologically and conceptually—is enormous.

Finally, the value of the computer in expanding fundamentally different models of intelligence, personality and cognition and, consequently, new paradigms of assessment is just beginning to be explored. As Hofer and Green (1985) have pointed out, dynamic, computational models of processing, reasoning, and other psychological phenomena have begun to emerge and receive evidence. Analogues of these developments in testing and assessment innovations has barely begun. An arena of particular relevance is that of diagnostic reasoning wherein the development of knowledge and inference based "expert" consulting systems holds considerable promise (see Gingerich, this volume).

In conclusion, there remains little doubt that computers are increasingly "in" our clinical practice – in our very language and conceptual models as well as more tangible forms such as the assessment tools reviewed in the prior paper (not to mention the multitude of administrative and daily agency functioning activities not addressed here). The need and opportunity is great for clinician involvement in the way of informed, proficient use of existing tools as well as through creative development and guidance of new computer-assisted innovations. Moreover, the responsibility for such involvement is great.

As advocates for their clients' welfare, practitioners have a responsibility to effectively *manage* the role and form of computers in clinical practice. To be effective managers (users, evaluators, developers) will require an integrated "literacy" in practice principals and realities as well as the relevant computer technology. Without this initiative, decisions will likely be rendered by those lacking in this more balanced perspective. As in any era of rapid change, the responsibility of individual practitioners is greater now than when tried and true guidelines could be relied on to guide policy and practice. Yet, with informed and tempered judgment, the new possibilities in assessment afforded through computer technology offer exciting and beneficial opportunities.

REFERENCES

Baer, W. S., Johnson, L. L., & Merrow, E. W. (1977). Government-sponsored demonstration of new technologies. *Science, 196,* 950-957.

Beresford, T., Law, D., Hall, R. C. W., Adduci, R., & Goggans, F. (1982). A computerized biochemical profile for detection of alcoholism. *Psychosomatics, 23*(7), 713-714, 719-720.

Block, J. (1965). *The challenge of response sets.* New York: Appleton-Century-Crofts.

Brooks, R. & Kleinmuntz, B. (1974). Design of an intelligent computer psycho-diagnostician. *Behavioral Science, 19,* 16-20.

Brown, D. T. (1984). Automated assessment systems in school and clinical psychology: Present status and future directions. *School Psychology Review, 13*(14), 455-460.

Buros, O. K. (1978). *The eighth mental measurements notebook.* Highland Park, NJ: Gryphon Press.

Butcher, J. N., Keller, L. S., & Bacon, S. F. (1985). Current developments and future directions in computerized personality assessment. *Journal of Consulting and Clinical Psychology, 53,* 803-815.

Byrnes, E. & Johnson, J. H. (1981). Change technology and the implementation of automation in mental health care settings. *Behavior Research Methods and Instrumentation, 13*(4), 573-580.

Carr, A. C., & Ghosh, A. (1983). Accuracy of behavioral assessment. *British Journal of Psychiatry, 142,* 66-70.

Carr, A. C., Ghosh, A., & Ancill, R. J. (1983). Can a computer take a psychiatric history? In M. Shepherd (Ed.), *Psychological medicine.* Cambridge: Cambridge Press.

Conklin, T. J. (1981). Computer applications in psychiatry workshop. In H. F. Heffeinan (Ed.), *Proceedings: The fifth annual symposium on computer applications in medical care.* New York: Institute of Electrical and Electronics Engineers, pp. 370-375.

Craig, T. J. (1984). Overcoming clinicians' resistance to computers. *Hospital and Community Psychiatry, 35*(2), 121-122.

Drazen, E. L. & Seidl, F. J. (1984). Implementation monitoring: A critical step towards realizing benefits from hospital information systems. In G. S. Cohen (Ed.), *Proceedings of the eighth annual symposium on computer applications in medical care.* New York: Institute of Electrical and Electronics Engineers.

Duthie, B. (1984). A critical examination of computer-administered psychological tests. In M. D. Schwartz (Ed.), *Using computers in clinical practice.* New York: The Haworth Press.

Erdman, H. P. (1983). *A comparison of computer consultation programs for primary care physicians: Impact of decision making model and explanation capability.* Unpublished doctoral dissertation, University of Wisconsin-Madison.

Farrell, A. D. (1984). When is a computerized assessment system ready for distribution? Some standards for evaluation. In M. D. Schwartz (Ed.), *Using computers in clinical practice.* New York: The Haworth Press.

Fowler, R. D. (1985). Landmarks in computer-assisted psychological assessment. *Journal of Consulting and Clinical Psychology, 53*(6), 748-759.

Geiss, G. (1983). Some thoughts about the future: Information technology and social work practice. *Practice Digest, 6*(3), 33-35.

Geiss, G. R. & Viswanathan, N. (Eds.), (1986). *The human edge: Information technology and helping people.* New York: The Haworth Press.

Gelernter, D. & Gelernter, J. (1984). Expert systems and diagnostic monitoring in psychiatry. In G. S. Cohen (Ed.), *Proceedings of the eighth annual symposium on computer applications in medical care.* New York: Institute of Electrical and Electronics Engineers.

Giannetti, R. A. & Klingler, D. E. (1980). A conceptual analysis of computerized mental health care systems. In J. B. Sidowski, J. H. Johnson, & T. A. Williams (Eds.), *Technology in mental health care delivery systems.* Norwood, NJ: Ables.

Graham, J. R. & Lily, R. S. (1984). *Psychological testing.* Englewood Cliffs, NJ: Prentice-Hall.

Greist, J. H. (1984). Conservative radicalism: An approach to computers in mental health. In M. D. Schwartz (Ed.), *Using computers in clinical practice.* New York: The Haworth Press.

Greist, J. H., Gustafson, D. H., Stauss, F. F., Rowse, G. L., Laughren, T. P., & Chiles, J. A. (1973). A computer interview for suicide-risk prediction. *American Journal of Psychiatry, 130*(12), 1327-1332.

Greist, J. H., Jefferson, J. W., Combs, A. M., Schou, M., & Thomas, A. (1977). The Lithium Librarion: An international index. *Archives of General Psychiatry, 134,* 456-459.

Greist, J. H., Klein, J. H., & Erdman, H. P. (1976). Routine on-line psychiatric diagnosis by computer. *American Journal of Psychiatry, 133,* 1405-1408.

Hammer, A. L. & Hile, M. G. (1985). Factors in clinicians' resistance to automation in mental health. *Computers in Human Services, 1*(3), 1-25.

Harris, W. G. (1984, August). Use of computer based test interpretation: Some possible guidelines. In J. D. Matarazzo (Chair), *Computer-based test interpretation: Prospects and problems.* Symposium conducted at the annual convention of the American Psychological Association, Toronto, Ontario, Canada.

Hedlund, J. L., Vieweg, B. W., & Cho, D. W. (1985). Mental health computing in the 1980's: II. Clinical applications. *Computers in Human Services, 1*(2), 1-31.

Hofer, P. J. & Bersoff, D. N. (1984). *Standards for the administration and interpretation of computerized psychological testing.* Unpublished manuscript.

Hofer, P. J. & Green, B. F. (1985). The challenge of competence and creativity in computerized psychological testing. *Journal of Consulting and Clinical Psychology, 53,* 826-838.

Hoshino, G. (1981). Computers: Tool of management and social work practice. *Administration in Social Work, 5*(3-4), 5-10.

Johnson, J. H. (1979). Technology. In T. A. Williams & J. H. Johnson (Eds.), *Mental health in the 21st century* (pp. 157-165). Lexington, MA: D.C. Heath.

Johnson, J. H. (1984). An overview of computerized testing. In M. D. Schwartz (Ed.), *Using computers in clinical practice.* New York: The Haworth Press.

Johnson, J. H., Giannetti, R. A., & Williams, T. A. (1976). Computers in mental health care delivery: A review of the evolution toward interventionally relevant on-line processing. *Behavior Research Methods and Instrumentation, 8*(2), 83-91.

Johnson, J. H. & Johnson, K. N. (1981). Psychological considerations related to the development of computerized testing stations. *Behavior Research Methods and Instrumentation*, *13*(4), 421-424.

Johnson, J. H. & Williams, T. A. (1980). Using on-line computer technology to improve service response and decision-making effectiveness in a mental health admitting system. In J. B. Sidowski, J. H. Johnson, & T. A. Williams (Eds.), *Technology in mental health care delivery systems* (pp. 237-252). Norwood, NJ: Ablex.

Johnson, J. H., Williams, T. A., Giannetti, R. A., Klingler, D. E., & Nakashima, S. R. (1978). Organization preparedness for change: Staff acceptance of an on-line computer-assisted assessment system. *Behavior Research Methods and Instrumentation*, *10*, 186-190.

Johnson, J. H., Williams, T. A., Klingler, D. E., & Giannetti, R. A. (1977). Interventional relevance and retrofit programming: Concepts for the improvement of clinician acceptance of computer-generated assessment reports. *Behavior Research Methods and Instrumentation*, *9*, 123-132.

Klonoff, H. & Clark, C. (1975). Measuring staff attitudes toward computerization. *Hospital and Community Psychiatry*, *24*(12), 823-825.

Levitan, K. B., Willis, E. A., & Vogelgesang, J. (1985). Microcomputers and the individual practitioner: A review of the literature in psychology and psychiatry. *Computers in Human Services*, *1*(2), 65-84.

Matarazzo, J. M. (1983, July 22). Computerized psychological testing. *Science*, *221*, 323.

McDermott, P. A. (1980). A computerized system for the classification of developmental, learning, and adjustment disorders in school children. *Education and Psychological Measurement*, *40*, 761-768.

Miller, D. A., Johnson, J. H., Klingler, D. E., Williams, T. A., & Giannetti, R. A. (1977). Design for an on-line computerized system for MMPI interpretation. *Behavior Research Methods and Instrumentation*, *9*(2), 117-122.

Moreland, K. L. (1985). Validation of computer-based test interpretations: Problems and prospects. *Journal of Consulting and Clinical Psychology*, *53*(6), 816-825.

Morf, M. E., Alexander, P., & Fuerth, T. (1981). Fully automated psychiatric diagnosis: Some new possibilities. *Behavior Research Methods and Instrumentation*, *13*(4), 413-416.

Robins, L. N., Helzer, J. E., Ratcliff, K. S., et al. (1982). Validity of the Diagnostic Interview Schedule, Version II: DSM-III diagnoses. *Psychological Medicine*, *12*, 855-870.

Ropper, A. H., Griswold, K., McKenna, D., & Sander, D. (1981). Computer-guided neurologic assessment in the neurologic intensive care unit. *Heart-Lung*, *10*(1), 54-60.

Sampson, J. P. & Pyle, K. R. (1983). Ethical issues involved with the use of computer-assisted counseling, testing, and guidance systems. *Personnel and Guidance Journal*, *61*(5), 283-286.

Schwartz, M. D. (1981). Interactive video in medicine: Tape or disc? In H. G. Hefferman (Ed.), *Proceedings of the fifth annual symposium on computer ap-*

plications in medical care. New York: Institute of Electrical and Electronics Engineers.

Schwartz, M. D. (1984). Interactive video. *Computers in Psychiatry/Psychology*, *6*(1), 7-13.

Skinner, H. A. & Allen, B. A. (1983). Does the computer make a difference? Computerized versus face-to-face versus self-report assessment of alcohol, drug, and tobacco use. *Journal of Consulting and Clinical Psychology*, *51*(2), 267-275.

Space, L. G. (1981). The computer as psychometrician. *Behavior Research Methods and Instrumentation*, *13*(4), 595-606.

Spitzer, R. L. (1983). Are clinicians still necessary? *Comprehensive Psychiatry*, *24*(5), 400-411.

Stout, R. L. (1983). New approaches to the design of computerized interviewing and testing symptoms. *Behavior Research Methods and Instrumentation*, *13*, 436-442.

Turkington, B. (1984, January). The growing use and abuse of computer testing. *APA Monitor*, *15*(1), 7.

Weiss, D. J. (1985). Adaptive testing by computer. *Journal of Consulting and Clinical Psychology*, *53*, 774-789.

Zachary, R. A. & Pope, K. S. (1984). Legal and ethical issues in the clinical use of computerized testing. In M. D. Schwartz (Ed.), *Using computers in clinical practice*. New York: The Haworth Press.

A First Order Markov Model for Use in the Human Services

Alvin O. Korte

KEYWORDS. Markov chains, markov processes, matrix algebra, market share analysis, operations research, program evaluation, research, administrative process, computer programs

SUMMARY. Markov processes have found a variety of uses in human services administration, evaluation, program and policy research. The models are concerned with the movement of entities or persons through finite states or conditions, the course of a disease and the movement of persons in various states in population change problems. The possibility of using the computer to link costs factors in levels of psychiatric and medical care as persons move through a system makes the first-order Markov process a potentially powerful tool in the administration of human programs.

Given the continued scarcity of fiscal and human resources it is incumbent upon the social services administrator or program evaluator to think in terms of efficient use of scarce resources in order to maximize their impact on social services to those in need. Many operation research (OR) models follow the resource optimization concept and can be adapted to human service program applications.

Dr. Alvin O. Korte is a Professor of Social Work at New Mexico Highlands University at Las Vegas, NM where he has taught for the last 15 years. Dr. Korte teaches research methods, human behavior, and aging with a special interest in Hispanic aging. His recent interest is in the applications of operations research models to human services organizations.

299

A recent volume collects diverse examples of OR models useful in the health care field (Kwak, Schmidt and Schniederjans, 1984).

This paper will examine one application of the first-order finite Markov process using an available computer program. The model will be discussed in terms of data requirements, available software, literature illustrating its use in human services programs and the minimal mathematics required for conceptual understanding and implementation.

OPERATIONS RESEARCH AND HUMAN SERVICES

Operations research was used during World War II to solve problems of logistics, scheduling, allocation of resources and planning. After the war the uses of operations research found many applications in business. Only recently has there been an effort to encourage its use by the National Institute of Mental Health in the administration of mental health programs and services (Kessler, 1981a,b).

Operations research is concerned with (1) sequencing of jobs; (2) allocation of scarce staff and material resources; (3) routing of products and the development of routes to minimize cost and time; (4) replacement of worn out equipment; (5) inventorying of items and reordering of items and supplies; (6) queuing, for example, how many persons who are waiting for some service can actually be served; (7) competitive problems as when two or more resources are available for investments; and (8) search problems. The latter involves the retrieval of information for decision making. In each case the objective is to reduce or minimize the cost in time or money associated with collecting data to reduce errors (Gillette, 1976:3-5).

The operations research model formulates the resources problem much like the research cycle concept used in traditional empirical research. A composite listing from two sources (Gillette, 1976:2; Cooper, Bhat and LeBlanc, 1977:9) follows:

(1) Formulate the problem; (2) Construct the model; (3) Develop a solution to the problem; (4) Test the model; and (5)

Implement the solution. Generally operations research models are adjuncts in the administrative decision process providing another facet of information.

PREREQUISITES

There are some fundamental prerequisites needed in order to understand the nature of the type of Markov model to be covered in this paper. Matrix algebra concepts form the basis of much of the needed prerequisite mathematics. A matrix is a rectangular array of numbers arranged into rows and columns and classified according to the number of rows and columns. Thus a 3 by 3 matrix has three rows and three columns. A matrix with one row and three columns is called a row vector in some notations. Matrices need to be identified in terms of their characteristics as square, symmetrical, diagonal, correlational, transition, zero, and identity. Additionally, there is a need to understand concepts of scalar multiplication and certain proofs involving the multiplication of matrices or the multiplication of a matrix by its inverse to obtain an identity matrix.

Searle (1982) provides much of the needed mathematics and conceptual development for a better understanding of the basic concepts and operations with matrices. Operations with matrices cannot be simply taken for granted because although ". . . familiar concepts in the algebra of numbers do and should motivate us to consider analogous ideas and techniques for the algebra of matrices, we should not accept their validity without careful verification" (Gilbert and Koehler, 1984:161). Matrix operations such as addition, subtraction, multiplication or finding the inverse of a matrix can be performed on desktop computers using a variety of available BASIC programs such as those found in Golden (1975) or in Poole and Borches (1979).

The Markov process is a potentially powerful tool in planning and evaluation of some types of human services programs. A probabilistic, mathematical tool that describes behavior of certain types of finite systems over time can model the flow of persons or entities between various states or conditions in terms of the probabilities of an entity moving from one state to another over time (Drachman,

1981:95). In human service terms, "states" can be the movement of patients between levels of care or discrete situations.

A BRIEF REVIEW OF USES

Various types of Markov processes can be used to model myriads of applications in the human services. Outside the human services, Markov models have found uses in market share analysis in business (Draper and Nolin, 1964) and in assessing water policy options in a water conservancy district (Dallenbach and George, 1978). Within the human services a variety of applications exist. Meredith (1973) studied the movement of geriatric patients through several levels of care in state hospital wards. A similar application can be found in a study of the exit of mental hospital patients through transition living to community living (Drachman, 1981). Meredith (1976) also evaluated three types of education programs and their effectiveness in serving the mentally retarded in a hospital. Eyman, Tarjan and McGunigle (1967) evaluated the transition probabilities of progress of mentally retarded school patients versus non-school patients along a "desirable-undesirable" continuum.

In sociology the Markov chain has been used to study social mobility processes (Spilerman, 1972). In the health care area Markov analysis can be used to study the course of a disease or the progress of patients following a medical event. One project evaluated events following induced abortion (Schatman and Hogue, 1976); another studied the recovery of coronary patients (Thomas, 1968).

In other diverse areas, Markov processes were used to research career development (Gribbons, Halperin and Lohnes, 1966), the epidemiology of mental diseases (Marshall and Goldhamer, 1955), the prediction of the number of elderly requiring various levels of long term care services (Navarro, 1969), and finally in the ingress and egress of persons from public welfare (Gilbert and Koehler, 1984). In the clinical area some attention has been directed in the study of husband and wife interactions and behaviors (Gottman and Notarious, 1978). Rausch (1972) has used Markov models to simulate aggressive intergroup behavior of adolescents and to predict interactional outcomes.

AN EXAMPLE FROM MARKET SHARE ANALYSIS

Despite wide application in business and in industry many OR models need to be adapted for use in the human services. Market share analysis refers to one type of application of the Markov chain in which the marketing researcher is interested in which brand the customer is more likely to purchase the next time, or in future time periods. Translating an example from Shamblin and Stevens (1974) into a human service context provides a way of studying the problem. Suppose that a client can choose one of three services, A, B or C. The next service choice the client makes will be controlled by the present choice. Steps occur each time a new choice is made. There are three finite states in the system, the choices of A, B or C. The system can be in the present time or $n = 0$, the next possible outcome or time as $n = 1$, and the outcome or time after next or $n = 2$ and so on. The present system can be represented at time $n = 0$ and by the three states, S1, S2 or S3 or

State	Description of system
S1	Choice of Service A
S2	Choice of Service B
S3	Choice of Service C

At the next time period $n = 1$ (a period of five years), the client can decide to choose the same service, or change to either of the other two services. This new system can be represented by

Present purchase ($n=0$)	Next purchases ($n=1$) at the end of five years		
	% choosing A	% choosing B	% choosing C
A	40	30	30
B	20	50	30
C	25	25	50

The above table represents an assumed probability that a client who presently uses service A (S1) will use service A, B or C at the next time of choice. Similarly the table provides information on any of the other states (beginning with B and changing to A, remaining with B or changing to C or if starting at C then changing to A or B or remaining with C). The system now has six states representing all the possible moves or steps among states. The information can be rewritten as a table of probabilities called a transition matrix, denoted by P.

			To State		
			A (S1)	B (S2)	C (S3)
	From	A (S1)	.40	.30	.30
P =	State	B (S2)	.20	.50	.30
		C (S3)	.25	.25	.50

Transitions matrices may be derived from frequency tables. Each element in the frequency table is divided by the row total so that the row probabilities sum to exactly 1.00 or 100 percent. Each element in the transition matrix must be a probability ranging between 1 and 0. Two mathematical assumptions must be made in order to compute transition states. It is assumed that the probability that an individual moves from one step at time T to another step at T + 1 depends only on his location at time T and not on his location at earlier times. The second assumption holds that transition probabilities do not change over time, that is the probability of going from one step to another is independent of the current step number. If both assumptions are met the process is called a first-order stationary Markov process or chain (Drachman, 1981:95; Gillette, 1976: 565-566). It is possible to determine the probability of an outcome after n steps, given some specified starting state S(i) (Shamblin and Stevens, 1974:56-57). The probabilities associated with change in some future states in a population problem is taken up in the next section.

AN EXPANDED EXAMPLE

Human services planning can be improved if population mobility is well understood. Suppose that an area has a population of 150 thousand living in one of three states, 60,000 in cities, 48,000 in suburbs and 42,000 in rural areas. A row vector, called an initial vector, termed P identifies the original locations of the 150,000 persons, in cities, suburbs and rural areas. In this example the initial vector is a row matrix or vector having one row and three columns corresponding to the three states and presents the initial population distribution below:

	Cities,	Suburbs,	Rural
P = [	60,000	48,000	40,000]

The row vector can be expressed as proportions or as initial probability terms respectively as:

$$P = [.400 \ .320 \ .280] \text{ or } P = [.40 \ .32 \ .28]$$

Assume that the following 3 by 3 matrix represents the shift in population in percentage terms at the end of a period of a year.

Population Shifts at the End of a Year

	To	City	Suburbs	Rural
	City	62%	34%	4%
From	Suburbs	19%	68%	13%
	Rural	17%	7%	76%

The same data can be represented as a transition matrix.

Population Shifts at the End of a Year

		To	City	Suburbs	Rural
$T^1 =$		City	62%	34%	.04%
	From	Suburbs	19%	68%	13%
		Rural	17%	.07%	76%

The transition matrices describe changes from one finite state to another. For example, those who began in the city and were still in the city at the end of a period of a year were 62 percent. The percent who moved from cities to suburbs is expressed as .34 or thirty-four and those who moved to rural areas from the city were four percent. Similar interpretations can be made for the other two classes. Another way to express the data is in probabilistic terms. One can ask, "What will be the probability that someone who began in a rural area at the beginning of a period will be in a city at the end of a year?" This can be expressed as a probability of .17 or the person has a .17 chance of being in the city if they begin initially in a suburb.

The product B = P(T*T) gives the population distributions at the end of two years. The matrix T is raised to the second power by a matrix multiplication and subsequently multiplied by P, the initial row vector as follows:

$$
\begin{array}{ccc}
P & & T^2 \\
B = [.40\ .32\ .28]\ * & &
\begin{array}{|ccc}
.456 & .445 & .099 \\
.269 & .536 & .195 \\
.248 & .234 & .594
\end{array}
\end{array}
$$

and solving for B we obtain B = [.338 .395 .268] indicating that from the initial population .338 or 33.8 percent will be in cities at the end of the second year, .395 or 39.5 percent will be in suburbs and 26.8 percent in rural areas.

The data was entered into the Dennis and Dennis (1986) computer programs which provided the following output.

HERE IS WHAT YOU ENTERED:

(0) NUMBER OF STATES = 3

Transition Matrix:

	1	2	3
(1)	.62	.34	.04
(2)	.19	.68	.13
(3)	.17	.07	.76

(4) TRANSITION (MARKET SHARE) ANALYSIS = Y
(5) NUMBER OF TRIALS OR PERIODS / 10

Beginning Vector or Matrix

	1	2	3
(6)	.4	.32	.28

OUTPUT SUMMARY:

TRANSITION MATRIX AFTER 1 TRIAL (PERIOD)

	1	2	3
1	.62	.34	.04
2	.19	.68	.13
3	.17	.07	.76

RESULTING VECTOR (MATRIX) — AFTER 1 PERIOD
.356   .373   .27

TRANSITION MATRIX AFTER 2 TRIALS (PERIODS)

	1	2	3
1	.456	.445	.099
2	.269	.536	.195
3	.248	.159	.594

RESULTING VECTOR (MATRIX) — AFTER 2 (PERIODS)
.338   .394   .268

A number of points can be made about the Markov program in Dennis and Dennis. One can input matrices as large as 12 by 12, that is twelve rows and twelve columns. In this case the matrix that was entered is a 3 by 3 matrix (NUMBER OF STATES = 3) at time n = 0. The computer program then sets up a three by three matrix in which the data is entered row by column until all the cells are filled. One is asked to verify the entries. The program will reject an entry if the row does not sum to 1.00. If a mistake has occured the program prompts one to change the row and its corresponding column. The program asks the user if a market analysis is called for. If the answer is Y for yes the program then asks for the initial vector. In row five (parenthesis) the program prompts for the number of times or periods to which the matrix T will be raised. In this case the matrix will be raised to the power of 2 or T multiplied by itself twice. The program can present as many period multiplications as are desired.

For our example the matrix T is raised to the second power to determine the composition of the population in two years. We learn that .456 or 45.6 percent will be in cities at the end of two years, while .445 or 44.5 percent will move from cities to the suburbs, while nine percent will move from cities to rural areas. Similar information can be gleaned for those that were in suburbs or in rural areas. The resulting vector gives the long run probabilities or numbers remaining in cities, in suburbs or in rural areas. Thus 33.8 percent will be in cities, 39.4 percent will be in suburbs and 26.8 percent will be in rural areas after two periods. We may ask, "What will be the population in thousands for those who move from cities to suburbs and to rural areas five years hence?'' The problem is again solved by raising the matrix to the fifth power then multiplied by P, the initial row vector. The Dennis and Dennis program provided the following output:

TRANSITION MATRIX AFTER 5 PERIODS:

	1	2	3
1	.338	.444	.219
2	.321	.422	.257
3	.312	.328	.360

RESULTING VECTOR (MATRIX) – 5 PERIODS:
.324   .404   .273

At the end of five years the initial row vector becomes B = [.325 .405 .270] indicating a loss of population in the cities (.325 percent or 47,917) persons and a subsequent increase in the suburbs, (.405 percent or 59,737) and a slight decrease to (.27 or 40,344 persons) in the rural areas. One advantage of the Dennis and Dennis program is that one can input the actual values in the initial vector, that is P = [60,000 48,000 40,000] and have the program return the values of 47,917, 59,737 and 40,344. The transition matrix raised to the fifth power is now:

	To	City	Suburbs	Rural
$T^5 =$	City	.338	.444	.219
From	Suburbs	.321	.422	.257
	Rural	.312	.328	.36

The above data illustrates a characteristic of some finite Markov chains. If the matrix is raised to increasingly higher powers a stage will ultimately be reached in which each value in each column will be the same. Thus for the first column the value for each row will reach .324, for the second column .404 and for the third column, .273. These states, called steady state probabilities mean that every state can be reached from every other state (possibly in a large number of states), and ". . . if the system can be in any given state on two consecutive steps, then the probability of being in any given state after a large number of steps is a constant. This constant is called the steady state probability for a given state" (Gillette, 1976:577). This data reached a steady state after raising the matrix 17 steps using the FORTRAN program in Gillette (1976). Similar results were achieved using the Markov program for the IBM PC in Dennis and Dennis (1986).

After 17 trials or periods the following matrix resulted.

	City	*Suburbs*	*Rural*
City	.324	.404	.273
Suburbs	.324	.404	.273
Rural	.324	.404	.273

Multiplying this stable matrix by the initial vector then results in the steady state probabilities of B = [.324,.404,.273], the same values as in the columns. For additional discussion on this characteristic of some Markov chains the reader is referred to Gilbert and Koehler (1984).

A study by Drachman (1981) illustrates the uses of many of these ideas to a typical human service situation. Drachman was concerned with the continuum of care for a group of chronic mental patients leaving a state hospital. Given that patients could move into and out of six different types of care during a 12-week period, Drachman was interested in predicting the number of mental patients who would be in the community 72 weeks hence or P to the power of six. Given an initial vector of P = [1, 0, 15, 8, 10, 53] for a total number of 87 patients at (1) the state hospital, (2) an inpatient unit, (3) a 24-hour group facility, (4) a 40-hour group facility, (5) a cooperative apartment and (6) in the community, respectively, Drachman obtained the following matrix for the 72nd week

	To:	State Hosp.	Inpatient Unit	24 Hr. Group	40 Hr. Group	Coop. Apt.	Community
	From:						
	St. Hosp	.1723	.0424	.2002	.0585	.0372	.4894
	Inpat.	.0678	.0359	.2032	.1010	.0600	.5323
	24 Hr	.0454	.0323	.2539	.1167	.0507	.5010
	40 Hr	.0548	.0330	.1256	.2373	.1046	.4447
$P^6 =$	Coop.	.0282	.0313	.1180	.0592	.2870	.4762
	Commu.	.048	.0374	.1758	.0548	.0758	.6073

In order to obtain estimates of the patients in the community 72 weeks hence the initial vector was multiplied by the elements in the community column. Drachman illustrates this by element-wise multiplication or $(1 \times .4894) + (0 \times .5323) + (15 \times .5010) + (8 \times .4447) + (10 \times .4762) + (53 \times .6073) = 48.71$ or 49 patients in the community at the end of the 72-week period. Expected and observed results were tested with a chi square test and according to the author the fit was excellent (Drachman, 1981: 100). The program was run on the Dennis and Dennis Markov program with similar results.

Drachman's interesting application discerns for the reader the possibility of determining similar estimates for the patients in the other care groups in the continuum of care. One of the applications of the model that makes it useful beyond predicting numbers of persons in various states at different time periods is the possibility of applying cost estimates for the care of persons in various care states. Anticipated costs per patient per month can be estimated by knowing the expected numbers of patients who will be in various types of living environments in the community. Meredith's (1973) study is a case in point. Meredith's study provides an example in which elderly pass through various wards in a hospital. Meredith not only provides a means of linking costs per state or the program's economic performance as well as accounting for the possibility of dying or leaving the system.

These types of Markov processes utilize a type of Markov chain which accounts for persons exiting the system by using "absorbing" states and requires a different mathematical approach than the one developed in these pages. Meredith's study of optimal training programs for the retarded also makes use of absorbing states as well as an analysis of the relative cost of the programs (Meredith, 1976). Both the Dennis and Dennis (1986) and Gilbert and Koehler (1984) computer programs allows for the use of absorbing states.

Some final notes concern the first-order Markov process and social systems concepts. It is to be observed that the first-order Markov chain fits concepts from social system theory rather well (Anderson and Carter, 1984). The ideas of steady states fits the discussion in Carter and Anderson. In the selection of states for model building, attention needs to be directed to selecting mutually exclusive and discrete states. Additionally it would seem that the selection of time periods for an analysis would depend on a thorough understanding of the system being modeled. Although not covered in this paper a further extension would be to examine social policy changes and its subsequent effects on number of persons who end up in various states (Meredith, 1973:610-611). This application of policy changes using Markov processes can be easily modeled on the computer programs discussed.

CONCLUSION

This paper has dealt with the simplest of Markov chains. Attention has been directed to the prerequisite understanding of some fundamental ideas in matrix manipulations. Knowledge of basic matrix operations is important not only in understanding Markov chain processes but to understand the means by which the computer solves for and predicts future states in the transition matrix. A basic understanding of matrix algebra helps in the understanding of other operations research models. A rich literature in the human services underscores the importance of and uses of first-order Markov processes. Computer programs for desktop computers means more flexibility in direct applications in program evaluation, research and as an adjunct in the administrative decision making process.

BIBLIOGRAPHY

Anderson, Ralph E. & Carter, Irl. *Human Behavior and the Social Environment A Social Systems Approach* (3rd Ed.). New York: Aldine Publishing Co. 1984.

Cooper, Leon. U., Bhat Narayan & LeBlanc, Larry J. (1977). *Introduction to Operations Research Models*. Philadelphia, Penn.: W. B. Saunders Company.

Dallenback, Hans G. & George, John A. (1978). *Introduction to Operations Research Techniques*. Boston, Massachusetts: Allyn and Bacon, Inc.

Dennis, Terry L. & Dennis, Laurie B. (1986). *Microcomputer Models for Management Science*. St. Paul, Minn.: West Publishing Company.

Drachman, David. (1981). "A Residential Continuum for the Chronically Mentally Ill." *Evaluation and the Health Professions.* 4 (1) 93-104.

Draper, Jean E. & Nolin, Larry H. (1964). "A Markov Chain Analysis of Brand Preferences." *Journal of Advertisement Research.* 4 (3), 33-38.

Eyman, R. K., Tarjan G. & McGunicle, D. (1967). "The Markov Chain as a Method for Evaluating Schools for the Mentally Retarded." *American Journal of Mental Deficiency*. 72, 435-444.

Gilbert, Gary G. & Koehler, Donald O. (1984). *Applied Finite Mathematics*. New York: McGraw-Hill Book Company.

Gillette, Billy E. (1976). *Introduction to Operations Research: A Computer Oriented Algorithmic Approach*. New York: McGraw Hill Book Co.

Gribbons, W. D., Halperin, S. & Lohnes, P. R. (1966). "Applications of Stochastic Models in Research on Career Development." *Journal of Counseling Psychology*. 13 (4), 403-408.

Golden, Neal. (1975). *Computer Programming in the BASIC Language*. New York: Harcourt Brace Jovanovich.

Gottman, John M. & Notarious, Cliff (1978). "Sequential Analysis of Observational Data Using Markov Chains." In P. Krawchowill (Ed.), *Single Subject Research Strategies for Evaluating Change*. New York: Academic Press, 237-284.

Kessler, Larry G. (Ed.). (1981a). *Operations Research and the Mental Health Service System (Vol. I). Report of Ad Hoc Advisory Group*. Washington, D.C.: U.S. Department of Health and Human Services, Public Health Service, ADAMHA, National Institute of Mental Health.

Kessler, Larry G. (Ed.). (1981b). *Operations Research and the Mental Health Service System (Vol. II). Critical Review and Annotated Bibliography*. Washington, D.C.: U.S. Department of Health and Human Services, Public Health Service, ADAMHA, National Institute of Mental Health.

Kwak, N. K., Schmitz, Homer H. & Schniederjans, Marc J. (Eds.). (1984). *Operations Research Applications in the Health Care Planning*. Lanham, Maryland: University Press of America.

Marshall, A. W. & Goldhammer, H. (1955). "An Application of Markov Processes to the Study of the Epidemiology of Mental Diseases." *Journal of American Statistical Association*. 50, 99-129.

Meredith, Jack. (1973). "A Markovian Analysis of a Geriatric Ward." *Management Science*. 19 (6), 604-612.

Meredith, Jack. (1976). "Selecting Optimal Training Programs in a Hospital for the Mentally Retarded." *Operations Research*. 24. October. 899-915.

Navarro, Vincent. (1969). "Planning Personal Health Services: A Markovian Model." *Medical Care*. May-June (Vol. VII). (3), 242-249.

Poole, Lpu. & Borchers, Mary. (1979). *Some Common Basic Programs*. (3rd. ed.) Berkeley, California, Osborne/McGraw Hill.

Rausch, H. L. (1972). "Process and Change A Markov Model for Interaction." *Family Process*. 11, 275-298.

Searle, Shayle R. (1982). *Matrix Algebra Useful for Statistics*. New York: John Wiley & Sons Inc.

Schactman, R. H. & Hogue, C. J. (1976). "A Markov Chain Model for Events Subsequent to Induced Abortion." *Operations Research*. 24, 916-932.

Causal Thinking and Computer Literacy

Charles McClintock

KEYWORDS. Causal thinking, cognitive heuristics, professional knowledge, computer literacy

SUMMARY. Professional practice in the human services often is based on implicit theories of causality regarding assessment of a problem and related interventions in a client's life. Complex applications of computing to this kind of professional activity require literacy about the underlying processes by which individuals make causal judgments. This paper presents a conceptual framework for understanding three components of causal thinking, the causal field, cues-to-causality, and causal theories, and their relationship to computing applications. For each component, several cognitive heuristics are described that can help individuals understand the components of causal thinking and link them to computer applications that might enhance the quality of professional practice.

Computer literacy is a useful form of knowledge for human service professionals, to the extent that it enhances their work skills. Computer applications might begin with simple and routine information tasks such as word processing or accounting in which no new knowledge is created, but efficiencies of operation are improved. At the other end of the scale are "intelligent" applications

---

Charles McClintock is Associate Professor in the Department of Human Service Studies, MVR-N136A, Cornell University, Ithaca, NY 14853-4401. His teaching and research are in the areas of organizational behavior, program evaluation and information management. Currently, he is doing research on tacit knowledge and causal reasoning in administrative and professional practice, and on how such knowledge is acquired through experiential learning.

that may involve complex improvisational episodes of professional practice, similar to what Schön (1983) refers to as "reflection-in-action," in which multiple definitions of problems and solutions are explored. Reflective practice is a significant antidote to the value conflict, uniqueness of circumstance, and ambiguity of causal interpretation that are common to professional-client interactions. The utility of computing and computer literacy for professional practice is shifting from an emphasis on efficiency in performing routine tasks to more complex cognitive applications, in which manipulating information enhances practitioner effectiveness and adds value to the work product (Strassman, 1985).[1]

Professional practice in the human services often involves complex assessment and intervention in a client's life in order to achieve a desired outcome: A social worker plans family counseling where child abuse has occurred; a teacher develops a tutoring program for underachieving students; an employer offers a child care program to employees to boost their productivity and reduce turnover and absenteeism; a doctor performs a battery of diagnostic tests for a possibly terminal patient. In each case these complex professional judgments are based on implied theories of causality in which certain factors are thought to produce undesirable effects, suggesting that interventions will change or counteract these negative causes. An important cognitive process for human service professionals is attributing causality for behavior and events, since these attributions underlie the means-ends relationship between interventions and their expected effects on client improvement and well-being.

Computing can be useful to many human service tasks that require complex or large scale information processing such as determining eligibility for service, case management, communications, obtaining reimbursement for services, budgeting, monitoring client progress and quality assurance, and program planning and evaluation (LaMendola, 1985). This paper will explore a different kind of application; namely, how computing can be of use to human service professionals to enhance their causal judgements about client problems and possible solutions.

First, it will be useful to place the role of causal interpretation in the larger context of cognitive perspectives on professional practice in human service settings. Following that, I will describe a framework for understanding the cognitive aspects of causal judgement. For each part of the framework I will present several cognitive heuristics and computing applications that could be used to enhance causal thinking (see Table 1 for an overview). The value of computing applications for each of these heuristics depends upon a prior understanding of the concepts of causal thinking. With respect to intelligent applications, computer literacy is only workable if the user is conversant with the underlying cognitive process.

COGNITION AND PROFESSIONAL PRACTICE IN HUMAN SERVICE SETTINGS

The role of causal thinking in professional practice is particularly important from the cognitive perspective on behavior in organizations (Schön, 1983; Sims & Gioia, 1986; Weick, 1979). In this view a critical unit of activity is the sense-making process in which causal interpretations represent an important kind of ambiguity commonly encountered in professional practice. Ambiguity is the product of the following kinds of conditions: (1) perceptions of problems and solutions are varied and often not explicit, (2) service outcomes are governed more by trial and error than by planned action, (3) the nature of the problems or work is often unclear or changing, (4) goals and causal processes are subject to change and multiple interpretation, and (5) objective standards for evaluation are generally lacking, forcing reliance on socially determined or value-based criteria for judging success (McCaskey, 1982).

The concepts of cognition, ambiguity and sense-making are especially significant for human service settings. Human services refer to those activities whose purpose is to ". . . maintain or improve the general well-being or functioning of people" (Hasenfeld & English, 1974, pg. 1). While it is possible to classify entire organizations as human services (e.g., schools, hospitals, social service agencies), many types of organizations contain human service activities. For example, administrative, marketing, personnel, planning, training and internal audit roles, with their emphasis on serving others, can be thought of as embodying human service responsibilities, regardless of the organizational setting (Eden, Jones, & Sims, 1983). Similarly, matrix and project management

Table 1. Overview of Causal Thinking, Cognitive Heuristics, and Computing
          Applications

Causal Thinking Processes	Cognitive Heuristics	Computing Applications
1. The causal field establishes a frame of reference for defining problems. A causal field identifies cause and effect variables, highlights dynamic causes from standing conditions, and focuses attention on relevant comparisons.	Metaphor Analysis Concept Maps Relational Algorithm	Text Editing Hypertext Outliners Structured Graphics Multidimensional Scaling
2. Cues-to-causality a. Covariation patterns among consensus, consistency, and distinctiveness information are used to make causal attributions.	Draw attention to under-represented patterns of information with hypothetical contingency tables and sampling distributions.	Statistical Analysis
b. The salience of a cause is determined by the temporal order, contiguity, and similarity of an effect.	Mapping Sentences	Decision Support Systems Expert Systems Artificial Intelligence
3. Causal theories reflect the implicit means-ends logic in definitions of human service problems and interventions. Causal loops are difficult to detect in implicit theories of causality.	Cause Maps	Structured Graphics and Drawing Statistical Analysis System Dynamics Simulations

structures in organizations, rely on the ability of professionals to make their specialized services useful among an interdisciplinary team; that is, professionals must treat each other as clients (Davis & Lawrence, 1977).

Hasenfield and English (1974, pg. 1-32) describe several distinctive attributes of human service tasks that highlight the importance of cognitive processes. First, human service professionals work with human beings as their "raw material." Interpersonal perceptions, moral judgment, social norms and status, and client motivation and autonomy are critical to the effectiveness of service treatments, and to relations between professionals and clients.

Second, the goals in human services are often value-laden, ambiguous and conflicting. For example, approaches to the treatment of juvenile delinquency will be seen by different segments of society as serving such varied purposes as personal growth, reform, control and prevention, or substitution for familial care and responsibility. A given human service encounter may also reflect the differing goals of client, professional, and organization, and a mixture of norms and standards from accrediting, advocacy, professional, or ideological groups. Finally, the "technology" of human service treatments or tasks is often indeterminant, due to variability in human characteristics, motivations and moods, the clarity of the outcomes that are sought, and the state of theory and knowledge about cause-effect relationships that will produce desired change.

Ambiguity can be healthy as well as vexing for professional practice. The nature of human service tasks highlights the importance of formative interpretations of causality that will foster experimental strategies of professional action (McClintock, 1986). This approach requires a balance between answering existing questions and raising new ones. Useful causal thinking will produce testable models, and also lead the human service professional to question the assumptions and structure of those models.

To summarize, the cognitive environment of ambiguity and sense-making in the human services is consistent with what Schön (1983) describes as the key challenge for effective professional practice. Schön's "reflective practitioner" is a professional who responds creatively to situations where novelty, ambiguity and conflicting values are the rule. This skill is dependent to a large extent on the ability to reason about the implicit theories of causality underlying professional action, and thus might be significantly improved with appropriate use of computer applications (Schweiger, Anderson, and Locke, 1985).

CAUSAL THINKING, COGNITIVE HEURISTICS AND COMPUTING APPLICATIONS

Causal thinking is used here to refer to *cognitive processes* by which individuals infer or assume causes. Causal judgement and its application in everyday life have received considerable attention within psychology, philosophy, sociology, statistics, health and law (Einhorn & Hogarth, 1986). Integrative models of causal thinking have emerged that combine the systematic and normative rules of causal inference dating to Kant and Hume, with current understanding of the cognitive bases of human inference in everyday judgment of causality. The framework described by Einhorn and Hogarth represents such an integrative effort. For this reason, as well as its underlying compatibility with Schön's description of the reflective practitioner, the Einhorn and Hogarth framework will be used to give an overview of three major components of causal interpretations: (1) the causal field, (2) cues-to causality, and (3) causal theories. For each component, heuristic activities and related computing applications are described that could be used to sharpen awareness of causal thinking that implicitly supports instances of professional practice.

THE CAUSAL FIELD

The causal field or frame of reference is an orienting concept in analyses of causal thinking. Defining the boundaries of a causal field determines which variables are perceived as possible causes, highlights dynamic causes from standing conditions and constraints, and focuses attention on alternative explanations.

The concept of the causal field embodies the basic distinction between figure and ground. Events that create change in a perceptual field are seen as figural against a set of standing or background conditions. For example, when a teacher examines students' knowledge, the variation in student performance typically is the only information available to the teacher and thus student ability is seen as the figural cause that stands out against the background conditions of the knowledge being tested. Changes in the perception of figure/ground relationships can be produced by introducing new information or highlighting already available information. Thus, to change a teacher's causal attribution that a student's low test score was caused by a lack of ability, one could provide information about student knowledge and skills that were not assessed by the test. The test then becomes the figural cause and its limitations are seen as the determinant of low scores against the background of student attributes.

Causal fields can be created by making comparisons, and in the human services, and computer-based information systems are often used to make comparisons among client groups, cohorts, agencies and time periods (James, Finch & Fanshel, 1985). The selection of a particular comparison group has the effect of defining a causal frame of reference on a problem, and is at least implicitly related to making arguments about alternative causal explanations or other threats to the internal validity of a particular causal inference. For instance, in explaining the causes of child abuse, if one focuses on the causal effects of environmental conditions such as economic cycles, then it would be relevant to present comparisons showing that child abuse occurs twice as often by parents who experience episodic unemployment and three times as often in households with chronic unemployment, in contrast to families with greater economic self-sufficiency. A different set of comparisons, such as the frequency of child abuse between parents who themselves were and were not abused in childhood, changes the causal field to one in which personality and attitudes towards child rearing are causal against the background of family dynamics.

A different kind of shift in the causal field would be represented by showing that there is more official information available on families who have contact with public agencies. This kind of comparison suggests that previous explanations of child abuse are artifacts of differential knowledge about the lives of families of varying socio-economic status.

Causal fields for professional action can be formulated at aggregate levels of economic forces, social or family dynamics, or at more molecular levels of psychological functioning or physiological processes. Reducing a societal level explanation to one in which physiological processes are dominant does not negate the former, but it shifts the focus of causal explanation and thereby influences

the way in which solutions will be imagined and intervention undertaken.

Cognitive Heuristics and Computing Applications

Exploring alternative causal fields often requires experimentation
with new concepts and their interrelationships. Several cognitive
heuristics for conceptualizing alternative causal fields have been
described by McClintock (1987a) as follows:

(1) Analysis of metaphors can reveal alternative causal fields for
conceptualizing professional problems and programs (Schön,
1983). For instance, to understand the assumptions and implicit theories underlying hospice care for the terminally ill, professionals
could explore contrasting metaphors for medical intervention such
as curative vs. palliative care. Emphasis on the first metaphor highlights concepts such as disease and death of the terminally ill person, while the latter suggests a different avenue of causal inquiry
about processes of transition and continuity among the lives of family members (McClintock, 1987b).

(2) Concept maps are graphic representations of individual perceptions of how things (i.e., nouns) are related to each other (with
verbs, prepositions and conjunctions). Professionals can create diagrams of their practice settings by labeling important concepts (perhaps from the metaphor exercise) and connecting the concepts with
lines and verbal statements that describe their causal and relational
structure (Novak & Gowin, 1984). Variation among concept maps
stimulates discussion about the relative clarity and utility of different perspectives on the problem (e.g., societal to physiological factors that contribute to child abuse).

(3) Relational algorithms are syntax exercises that can be used to
identify unimagined relationships among concepts in a causal theory (Weick, 1979). To create a relational algorithm one begins with
a short statement of a problem (e.g., an agency strives to care for its
most needy clients while maintaining sufficient cash flow for financial solvency). Next, it is necessary to focus on two terms that represent a dilemma in the statement (e.g., care vs. cash flow). Relational language (e.g., by, over, while) are systematically varied
between the two terms and connotations noted. For instance, "care

by cash flow'' suggests that causal primacy of financial resources in agency success, whereas "care *while* cash flow" connotes the potential for complementary causality between the two concepts.

There are several kinds of computing applications that could be helpful to human service professionals in using these heuristics for exploration of alternative causal fields. Most obvious are text analysis programs. For instance, *text editing* programs provide the user with summaries of key words or phrases in terms of their frequency and contextual associations with other language. These applications could be used for metaphor analysis of agency documents such as policy and goal statements by listing linguistic associations for key concepts (e.g., curative and palliative care), or to review relational connections by listing the relative frequency of combinations of key terms (e.g., curative care — *and*, versus, *leads to, with* — palliative care).

Hypertext programs, especially those with tree diagramming capabilities, could be used for exploring the hierarchical structure of concept maps. Different groups such as administrators, service delivery staff and clients could be asked to organize a set of concepts in outline format that describe a particular service. Figure 1 shows an example of a concept map for a model of care for hospice services. These concepts were first organized with a hypertext outline program and the resulting tree diagram of the outline was then modified with an application for creating *structured graphics*. The concept map in Figure 1 is only one of several hierarchical and horizontal structures for thinking about the causal field of hospice services. For one group of stakeholders principles of care might be at the top of the hierarchy while for others particular outcomes would subsume many other concepts. Discussion of varying concept maps becomes a vehicle for more thorough analysis of alternative causal fields, which in turn can create new ways of framing problems and human service interventions.

Exploration of causal fields can also be done by *multidimensional scaling* computer applications. Trochim and Linton (1985) describe several multivariate procedures that can be used to calculate perceived similarity among many verbal descriptors of a human service problem or program. Individuals generate a set of items related to the program in question (e.g., its goals, barriers to effectiveness,

Figure 1: A Concept Map of a Model of Care for Hospice Services

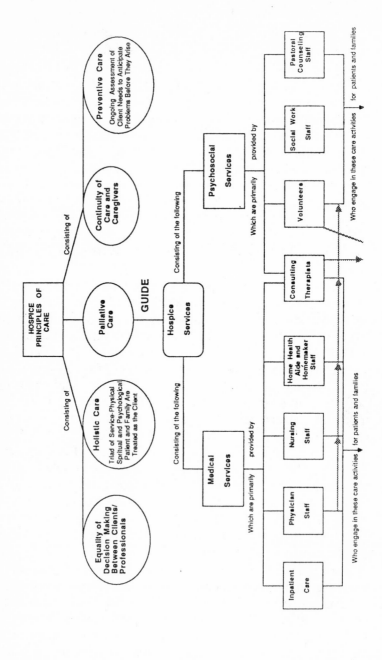

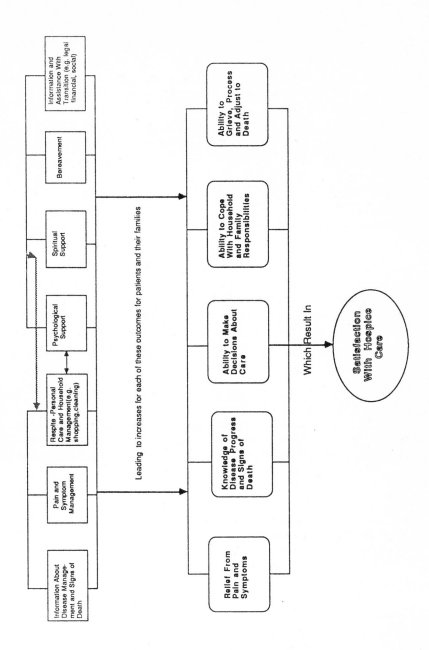

Information About Disease Management and Signs of Death

Pain and Symptom Management

Respite -Personal Care and Household Management(e.g. shopping,cleaning)

Psychological Support

Spiritual Support

Bereavement

Information and Assistance With Transition (e.g. legal financial, social)

Leading to increases for each of these outcomes for patients and their families

Relief From Pain and Symptoms

Knowledge of Disease Progress and Signs of Death

Ability to Make Decisions About Care

Ability to Cope With Household and Family Responsibilities

Ability to Grieve, Process and Adjust to Death

Which Result In

Satisfaction With Hospice Care

323

processes) and then sort them into meaningful groups. The computer program identifies concepts that represent groupings of individual descriptors. Users then can collapse and separate concepts as they create interpretations of the schematic concept maps that are generated from the scaling analysis.

Creating alternate causal fields sensitizes the human service professional to how problems are framed, and to the various ways in which important questions can be formulated. Asking insightful questions often takes one half the distance towards effective interventions. Next it is important to move from a conceptual to an empirical level of analysis, and to recognize how causal inferences are made from various informational cues.

CUES-TO-CAUSALITY

The second component in Einhorn and Hogarth's model of causal thinking, is referred to as cues-to-causality. The analysis of human inference regarding causal cues is too complex to portray in detail here, but it is possible to identify categories of cues that influence causal thinking.

Covariation

Patterns of covariation between a possible cause (X) and an observed effect (Y) are the most common focus in analysis of informal causal judgement. For instance, in Kelley's (1967) model of causal attribution there are three types of covariance information that are important to assess:

1. *consensus* addresses whether an effect was similar for a sample of different persons;
2. *consistency* examines whether an effect was similar across different circumstances, times or forms of the same cause;
3. *distinctiveness* questions whether an effect was similar across a sample of different causes.

For example, if a new method of teaching math produced increased math scores for most students (high consensus), when administered in different schools over time (high consistency), and different instructional programs (e.g., science) did not result in increased *math* scores (high distinctiveness), then the new teaching intervention would be interpreted as causing students to learn math. A different pattern of covariation might result in consensus and distinctiveness being low (e.g., the improvement in math scores only occurred with high ability students, and their scores improved from both science and math instruction). The resulting inference would favor high ability students as the cause of the outcome (i.e., their abilities caused them to improve regardless of the type of intervention). A covariance pattern showing high distinctiveness (improvement only occurred for math instruction), high consistency (across school settings) but low consensus (the effect occurred only for high ability students), would imply a causal interaction between the instructional program and a particular type of student.

Despite the apparent complexity in models of covariance analysis, evidence indicates that when provided with appropriate patterns of information, individuals can make use of covariance patterns in drawing normative causal interpretations, and for altering dysfunctional attributions (Fosterling, 1986). In addition these three sources of information can be found in many types of professional-client interaction, whenever there is discussion of what has caused an effect. Administrators might utilize consensus information to deflect negative attributions about themselves and to justify a particular decision as being the only possible response to a situational stimulus (e.g., given the situation anyone would have responded as I did); educators might use consistency information to demonstrate the causal efficacy of a remedial skills program (e.g., student achievement was increased in rural and urban settings, large and small schools, and across time periods or subject matter); therapists might use distinctiveness information to influence a client's self-attributions (e.g., your anxiety does not occur in all situations, but only increases when your authority is challenged).

At the same time, Nisbett and Ross (1980, Chapter 6) have identified numerous cognitive limitations and biases that impair causal interpretation (e.g., consensus information is often underused compared to distinctiveness and consistency). Limitations in everyday language also contribute to incomplete sampling of conditional or nonoccurring events [i.e., a cause (X) followed by no effect (Y), an effect (Y) preceeded by no cause (X), and no cause (X) with no effect (Y)]. For instance, clairvoyance and extra-sensory perception often are powerful causal candidates in situations where we mistakenly believe that a statistically unusual association between two events has occurred (e.g., a dream followed by a similar event). The absence of terminology in ordinary language limits the ability to describe other possible occurrences, such as a dream and no subsequent similar event, no dream and a subsequent significant event, or no dream and no significant event, and thus biases our thinking about alternative causal interpretations.

Temporal Order, Contiguity, and Similarity

Causal thinking is influenced by the temporal order of causes and effects, by their closeness in time and space, and by their physical or conceptual similarity. The salience of particular cues may create rigidity in causal thinking. Evidence suggests that people often inappropriately search for causes that are most available to memory, and that are similar in nature or scope to the attributes of the observed outcome (Nisbett & Ross, 1980, Chapters 2 and 3). This is especially problematic when causes are far removed in time, substance or size from the effects of concern. For example, given a serious event such as child abuse, cognitively it is easier to infer causality from immediately preceeding stressful events such as a child's tantrum, or events of similar character and severity in the abusers past such as a history of aggressive behavior. Many salient outcomes, however, are the result of repeated cycles of causal variables that do not resemble the qualities of the effect that eventually emerges. An instance of child abuse might be the end result of many cycles of a causal loop involving variables different from the eventual salient outcome of abuse, such as the parent's frustration in an endeavor followed by passivity and depression. Repeated cycles of this pattern, perhaps dating to childhood, combined with new circumstances of being a parent, could eventually result in aggression towards one even more helpless than the confused parent. Thus, it might be more appropriate to search for the antecedents of physical abuse in repeated cycles of passivity rather than aggressiveness.

Cognitive Heuristics and Computer Applications

There are two kinds of heuristics and related computer applications that could be helpful to human service professionals for interpreting cues-to causality.

(1) Typically, we are unable to cognitively analyze all possible combinations of covariation, thus it is helpful to draw our attention to unexamined covariance patterns. This process can be greatly facilitated with the use of *statistical analysis* programs. As a first step, the user can create hypothetical contingency tables of a cause (X) and its absence (no X) crosstabulated with a possible effect (Y) and the absence of that effect (no Y). Next, by focusing attention on past experiences that are represented by each cell in the contingency table, one can establish frequencies for the overlooked occurrences and calculate the resulting measures of association. Similarly, sampling simulations from artificial populations of known dimensions can reveal the spurious interpretations resulting from narrow or biased observational activities. The result of these activities will often be a recognition that the basic population distribution of an event or a type of client problem has been underestimated or otherwise misjudged (Nisbett & Ross, 1980).

(2) Complex patterns of cues-to-causality can be mapped into linguistic or decision tree formats in order to examine the consequences of lengthy or interactive if-then sequences (Canter, 1985). The following example illustrates a mapping sentence that could serve as the basis for understanding a temporal sequence of events:

The development of employer-sponsored family support programs for

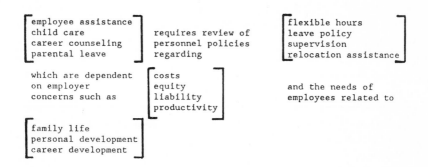

```
⎡employee assistance⎤                        ⎡flexible hours        ⎤
⎢child care         ⎥   requires review of   ⎢leave policy          ⎥
⎢career counseling  ⎥   personnel policies    ⎢supervision           ⎥
⎣parental leave     ⎦   regarding            ⎣relocation assistance ⎦

which are dependent    ⎡costs       ⎤
on employer            ⎢equity      ⎥         and the needs of
concerns such as       ⎢liability   ⎥         employees related to
                       ⎣productivity⎦

⎡family life          ⎤
⎢personal development ⎥
⎣career development   ⎦
```

Computer applications such as decision support systems, expert systems, and artificial intelligence can greatly expand the professional's ability to explore complicated sequences of cues for purposes of diagnosing problems and planning interventions. These applications share the common goal of supporting cognitive processes in which there is a need for extensive information search or the application of complex rules, classifications or inferences (Schoech et al., 1985; Vogel, 1985). Expert systems could incorporate the capacity to seek information on possible causes or diagnoses that are *dissimilar* to the observed effects, in addition to those that resemble them. Decision support systems could be programmed with simple inference rules to process the causal logic of covariance structures such as distinctiveness, consistency and consensus information. The computer application then could suggest causal conclusions based on analysis of data from management information systems describing patterns of effects across different human service programs, time periods and cohorts.

The analysis of cues-to-causality never occurs in a vacuum. Data are always interpreted within a perspective, even if it is not explicit. The final component of the framework focuses on how implicit theories influence causal thinking.

CAUSAL THEORIES

Cues-to-causality such as covariation, temporal order, or similarity often are linked together cognitively by an implicit theory about the relationships among a group of variables. The theory may be a simple linear chain of events, or a more complex model in which there are causal loops, indirect influences, interactive causal relations, or non-linear relationships. Varying employees' salary increases in order to influence their level of productivity is an example of a simple causal theory. More elaborate theories may be used to explain complex social problems such as delinquency, or to describe how professional interventions are expected to ameliorate those problems (Bickman, 1987). Implicit causal theories are similar to other cognitive structures that are common to professional-client interactions such as the following:

(1) Schemas about self and others in which clusters of attributes

are seen as characteristic of groups (e.g., social workers) or types of people (e.g., a passive-aggressive personality); (2) scripts that define the sequence of events that are expected to occur in a particular setting (e.g., the intake interview) or the implementation of a human service task (e.g., diagnosing an instance of child abuse) (Sims & Gioia, 1986, Chapter 1).

In professional practice settings, theories about client problems and interventions can be based on scientific research, expert opinion, and informal observation, but are more likely to evolve from "... maxims, parables, myths, fables, epigrams, allegories, well-known songs or novels, and anecdotes about famous people or personal acquaintances" (Nisbett & Ross, 1980, pg. 119). Although most causal theories are simplistic and implicit, they are important to understand since they often contribute to value conflict, ambiguity and uniqueness in how problems are defined and solutions imagined. Nisbett and Ross argue that when groups with opposing views are exposed to patterns of cues that should lead each group to question its own theory, often the result is to polarize opinions, "... with proponents of each side picking and choosing from the evidence so as to bolster their initial opinions" (pg. 171). On the other hand, there is considerable evidence that these limitations in causal thinking may be alleviated by explicating the varying implicit theories of the problem or intervention held by different individuals who are affected by it (Eden et al., 1983; Schön, 1983).

Bickman (1987) lists several additional reasons why clarification of implicit theories is useful in human service settings. Understanding the possible causal links among variables helps: (1) explain the intermediate causal processes that might have produced positive or negative outcomes; (2) facilitate generalizations to other human service problems and settings; (3) clarify if a failure to find positive effects is due to the theory underlying the intervention or the way the intervention was implemented; (4) determine whether the intervention is appropriately designed to address the causes of the problem; (5) clarify what variables might be influenced to improve outcomes; (6) identify unintended consequences; (7) guide data collection on critical indicators of progress; and (8) portray varying perceptions of different groups of stakeholders.

Although experts can have complex theories, most lay theories are simple, resistant to information that might lead to alternative interpretations, and often inappropriately applied to situations that have superficially similar stimuli (Nisbett & Ross, 1980, Chapter 6). Even among the formal theories of experts, however, there are few instances of causal loops and cyclical thinking (Axelrod, 1976). It is the cyclic or looping quality of many cause-effect relationships that creates ambiguity in causal interpretations. In causal loops, by definition, a factor can be seen as a cause and an effect. Thus, a symptom may be diagnostic of a previous cause (depression is diagnostic of previous frustration), and also seen as the cause of future symptoms similar to the prior cause (depression increases the likelihood of future frustration). Weick and Bougon (1986) describe additional problems in perceiving and acting on causal loops. First, individuals usually don't have feedback on their behavior with which to interpret reality in a cyclical fashion. There is, therefore, a tendency to think about causality in segmented linear episodes. Similarly, because behavior often occurs in many different settings, it is difficult to experience the longer term or cyclical consequences of numerous interrupted series of events. Finally, any causal loops may have relatively weak effects, or require embeddedness in an interactive nested fashion with other loops in order to have salient outcomes that might stimulate causal interpretation.

Cognitive Heuristics and Computer Applications

In order to portray and analyze implicit theories human service professionals can compose maps of perceived causal relationships. These maps are diagrams that show variables as points connected by directional arrows with plus or minus signs indicating whether the relationships are perceived to be positive or inverse correlations. Cause maps can be developed from document analysis, interview and observation, or questionnaires (Weick & Bougon, 1986). Figure 2 shows a simple map of causal loop representing a problem in health care costs (McClintock, 1987). Structured graphics and drawing applications can be used to portray individual cause maps or those based on the consensus of a group. The map then can function as a heuristic to complicate and test interpretations of a particular ''theory'' and its implications for intervention. For in-

Figure 2: A Cause Map of a Problem in Health Care Costs

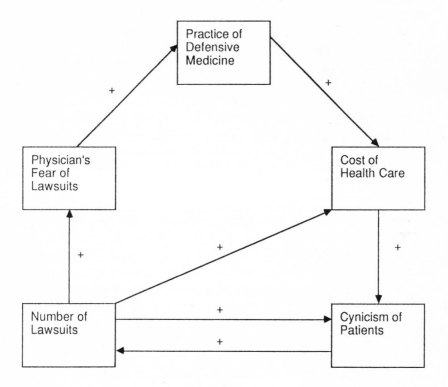

stance, Figure 2 could be used to explore the feasibility of the following action alternatives:

1. Reverse the causal direction between two variables: The number of lawsuits causes the level of patient cynicism.
2. Change the sign of a causal relationship: An increase in the number of lawsuits decreases physician fear.
3. Interrupt causality: Physician fear has no effect on defensive medicine.
4. Create variability in the direction of the relationship: Sometimes cynical patients file lawsuits, but as the number of lawsuits increases, patient cynicism is assuaged.
5. Remove a variable: Prohibit lawsuits against physicians.

6. Intensify or moderate a relationship: Physicians deliberately cost account defensive medicine practices which immediately leads to a significant increase in health care expenses; or, because of new cost containment regulations, defensive medicine has only a modest effect on costs.
7. Create another causal relationship that nullifies an undesirable effect: The number of lawsuits triggers a limit on the size of awards, which reduces physician fear.
8. Establish curvilinear relationships. Cynicism leads to lawsuits to the point where they become burdensome to patients, which leads to a search for alternative forms of care and a decline in lawsuits.

In addition to portraying cause maps with *computer graphics, statistical analysis* applications can be employed in a variety of ways. First, calculating simple frequencies of interconnections can be used to determine which variables are perceived as causes and which as effects. Elements that have more arrows outgoing from them are primarily causal or independent variables while those with more incoming arrows are primarily effect or dependent variables. The elements with comparable numbers of incoming and outgoing arrows are interdependent variables, and they have special significance due to their multiple causal connections. Alternatively through matrix operations one can analyze the strength of causal paths between any two variables by calculating the number of direct and indirect links between them. Finally, the rank ordered importance of variables can be determined by summing the frequency of their incoming and outgoing paths.

As discussed above, causal theories may have repeating cycles or loops that are difficult to identify. The long term effects of causal loops also are elusive since longitudinal observation often is necessary to identify significant outcomes. *System dynamics simulations* can be of help with these problems (Richardson & Pugh, 1981). System dynamics simulations are mathematical models that emphasize causal or feedback loops; that is, chains of causal connections that recycle back to a point of origin. These simulations represent a methodology for understanding interactive causal influence among many variables, by defining mathematical relationships among them that change their values over repeated cycles of the causal loops in the model. This kind of computing application is particularly useful because it performs more calculations than can be done mentally, shows the effects of multiple calculations on specific variables of interest, and demonstrates how variables influence each other over time. Simulations also allow one to explore assumptions about which variables are of critical importance to program or client outcomes of interest. This exploration can be done in several ways; (1) for instance by a sequential process of changing the range of values on selected variables, running the simulation, and noting the impact on outcomes of interest; or (2) by changing the mathematical relationships between variables. These activities constitute a kind of sensitivity analysis that identifies those variables that are likely to be most important to a desired outcome, and therefore that should be thoroughly examined in relation to professional intervention. System dynamics simulations allow the professional to create different models of a program, and because they can be run over any time frame, to explore multiple future scenarios.

CONCLUSION

If computer literacy is to make a difference in the effectiveness of human service professionals, it must be applied to more complex tasks such as causal thinking. The process of causal interpretation is one critical point at which computing can have a significant influence on human service practice, because of the direct implications of causality for the means-ends relationships that characterize professional intervention. The potential value of complex computing applications depends on the prior understanding of the processes that are being enhanced. This paper has presented a framework for understanding the process of causal thinking as it might apply to a variety of human service tasks, and described how computing applications could enhance several cognitive heuristics for defining problems and imagining solutions.

NOTE

1. A common definition of information is to distinguish it from data (Schoech, 1982, Chapter 2). Data are symbols (words, images, numbers) that represent events, conditions or objects. Data become information and acquire "value"

when they capture cognitive attention, are given meaning and utilized for some interpretive, analytic or communicative purpose. The term information will be used more often in this paper, due to the emphasis on complex and interpretive applications of computing for professional practice.

REFERENCES

Axelrod, R. (1976). *The structure of decision: The cognitive maps of political elites.* NJ: Princeton University Press.

Bickman, L. (1987). The functions of program theory. In L. Bickman (Ed.), *Using program theory in evaluation: New directions for program evaluation.* Vol. 33. San Francisco: Jossey-Bass.

Canter, D. (1985). *Facet theory: Approaches to social research.* New York: Springer-Verlag.

Davis, S. M., & Lawrence, P. R. (1977). *Matrix.* Reading, MA: Addison-Wesley.

Eden, C., Jones, S., & Sims, D. (1983). *Messing about in problems: An informal structured approach to their identification and management.* Elmsford, NY: Pergamon.

Einhorn, H. J. & Hogarth, R. M. (1986). Judging probable cause. *Psychological Bulletin*, 99, 2-19.

Fosterling, F. (1986). Attributional conceptions in clinical psychology. *American Psychologist*, 41, 275-285.

Hasenfield, Y. & English, R. A. (1974). Human service organizations: A conceptual overview. In Y. Hasenfield & R. A. English (Eds.), *Human service organizations.* Ann Arbor, MI: University of Michigan Press.

James, P., Finch, S. J., & Fanshel, D. (1985). Organizing routinely collected computerized data bases for evaluations of social care systems. *Computers in Human Services*, 1, 27-46.

Kelley, H. H. (1967). Attribution theory in social psychology. In D. Levine (Ed.), *Nebraska symposium on motivation.* Vol. 15. Lincoln, NE: University of Nebraska Press.

La Mendola, W. F. (1985). The future of human service information technology: An essay on the number 42. *Computers in Human Services*, 1, 35-50.

McClintock, C. C. (1986). Toward a theory of formative evaluation. In M. W. Lipsey & D. S. Cordray (Eds.), *Evaluation studies review annual.* Vol ll. Beverly Hills, CA: Sage.

McClintock, C. C. (1987a). Conceptual and action heuristics: Tools for the evaluator. In L. Bickman (Ed.), *Using program theory in evaluation: New directions for program evaluation.* No. 33. San Francisco: Jossey-Bass.

McClintock, C. C. (1987b). Systems dynamics simulations; Clarifying complex causal dynamics. Paper presented at the American Evaluation Association, Boston, MA.

McCaskey, M. B. (1982). *The Executive Challenge: Managing Change and Ambiguity.* Marshfield, MA: Pittman.

Nisbett, R., & Ross, L. (1980). *Human inference: Strategies and shortcomings of social judgement*. Englewood Cliffs, NJ: Prentice-Hall.

Novak, J. D., and Gowin, D. B. (1984). *Learning how to learn*. Cambridge, England: Cambridge University Press.

Richardson and Pugh (1981). *Introduction to system dynamics modeling with DYNAMO*. Cambridge, MA: MIT Press.

Schoech, D. (1982). *Computer use in human services: A guide to information management*. New York: Human Sciences Press.

Schoech, D., Jennings, H., Schkade, L. L., Hooper-Russell, C. (1985). Expert systems: Artificial intelligence for professional decisions. *Computers in Human Services*, 1, 81-115.

Schön, D. A. (1983). *The reflective practitioner: How professionals think in action*. New York: Basic Books.

Schweiger, D.M., Anderson, C.R., & Locke, E.A. (1985). Complex decision making: A longitudinal study of process and performance. *Organizational behavior and human decision processes*, 36, 245-272.

Sims, H. P., Jr., Gioia, D. A., & Associates (1986). *The thinking organization: Dynamics of organizational social cognition*. San Francisco: Jossey-Bass.

Strassman, P. A. (1985). *Information payoff: The transformation of work in the electronic age*. New York: The Free Press.

Trochim, W. M. K., & Linton, R. (1985). Conceptualization for planning and evaluation. *Evaluation and Program Planning*, 9, 289-308.

Vogel, L. H. (1985). Decision support systems in the human services: Discovering limits to a promising technology. *Computers in Human Services*, 1, 67-80.

Weick, K. E. (1979). *The social psychology of organizing*. Reading, MA: Addison-Wesley.

Weick, K. E., & Bougon, M. (1986). Organizations as cognitive maps: Charting ways to success and failure. In H. P. Sims, Jr., & D. A. Gioia (Eds.), *The thinking organization: Dynamics of organizational social cognition*. San Francisco: Jossey-Bass.

Conclusion

This volume was designed to provide the reader with an understanding of computer literacy in human services. Toward this end we have contributed a definitional framework, a discussion of computer literacy issues, and a broad array of examples that exemplify this body of knowledge.

It is apparent from a reading of this work that computers will have a strong influence on the future understanding and practice of human services. The specific nature of this change will, in many ways, be determined by those who participate in the use of computers in human services. Our hope is that all human service professionals will assume majority status as users. Thus, we dedicate this publication to all the human service professionals who contribute to the development of computer literacy in human services.

R.R.
T.H.